EBURY PR[ESS]

...NDING YOUR BALANCE

...ar is a consultant gynaecologist at Breach Candy, PD ...Holy Family hospitals in Mumbai, with a long-standing ... to women's health and rights. Having been in clinical practice for over thirty years, he has a vast experience of caring for women at every-life stage. A gold medallist at every postgraduate examination, he was awarded the FRCOG in acknowledgement of his support of women's health. He has edited fifteen books, and written over 110 chapters and scientific papers. He is a board member of the Guttmacher Institute and the Centre for Catalyzing Change, a technical adviser to the SEAR WHO and co-chair of the medical advisory panel FPAI. He was the secretary general of the National Federation of Obstetrics and Gynecology, and president of the Mumbai Society. He served FIGO as the scientific chair of the World Congress of Gynecology in Rio de Janeiro. With a keen interest in high-risk pregnancy, endoscopy, contraception, induced abortion and midlife care, he considers his practice of medicine to be a blend of science and art, complemented by his love of reading, music and sketching.

Shonali Sabherwal is India's first celebrity macrobiotic nutritionist and gut health expert. She uses food as medicine and works to strengthen the gut, with focus on immunity. It is rare that one gets a combination of a nutritionist and a chef in one person. Besides this, she has been trained in the art of 'Oriental organ facial diagnosis', and her advice stems from analysing organ imbalances first and then prescribing a diet plan. She complements this by combining Ayurvedic philosophy with the macrobiotic approach. She has worked for twenty years across more than fifty ailments, with over 8000 clients, 1000 articles in leading publications and 200 workshops. She has a presence in over thirty-five countries and is the recipient of the Times of India Woman Entrepreneur Award 2019 and the Vogue Award for the Best Nutritionist 2020. She is the author of the bestsellers *The Beauty Diet*, *The Love Diet* and *The Detox Diet*, and, most recently, of *Vipassana: The Timeless Secret to Meditate and Be Calm*. She also has a podcast called *Soul Food Conversations* on Audible by Amazon.

'This book comes to you from one of the best doctors in the field of women's health and someone who has been with me in my journey personally. As a woman myself, I understand how important knowledge about our own body is during the years we start experiencing different emotions triggered by changes in our body. This book will be a bible for generations and a reference manual for women on how to tackle all the issues we go through in our younger years leading to perimenopause. Shonali Sabherwal has added a totally holistic approach with her nutritional and lifestyle knowledge, and this makes the book a complete health manual for women'—Rani Mukerji, actor, philanthropist, mother, wife and daughter

'I often joke that we do get more comfortable in our skin as we age largely because our skin is also not as tight as it once used to be. Ageing and physical transitions are inevitable, but the more informed we are, the easier it gets. This book, by the brilliant Dr Nozer Sheriar and Shonali Sabherwal, is a buoy we can all hold on to, as we bob along hormonal waves and the occasional ocean of night sweats' —Twinkle Khanna, author, columnist and designer

'This book is an urgent and important intervention. The woman's body goes through many changes during perimenopause, and it can be debilitating in some cases. Knowing better always helps us do better. And who better to help than two doctors who are the best in women's health'—Dia Mirza, actor, producer and UN goodwill ambassador

'Women's health statistics in our country are shocking, and this will only change when more women prioritize their health and get educated on important health conditions. This book is an important tool for women to help them do exactly this. It is an easy read, yet full of essential information and facts, by two incredible experts. I am sure that this book will equip many women to take charge of their health'—Namita Thapar, entrepreneur, business leader and media personality

'For women, who now spend a large part of their lives post menopause this book is the perfect resource. It combines a guide to a healthy lifestyle with a presentation of the latest evidence-based medical developments in menopause care. Kudos to Shonali and Nozer for writing this must-read: a 360-degree approach to understanding and managing perimenopause'—Prof. Chitaranjan Purandare, gynaecologist and postgraduate teacher, and former president, FIGO, FOGSI and MOGS

'A beautiful blend of an in-depth understanding of evidence-based and holistic medicine pertaining to menopause. The book allows the reader to choose topics to suit her individual needs and beliefs. Well done, Shonali and Nozer'—Dr Nadeem Rais, endocrinologist, researcher and master clinician

'*Finding Your Balance* is a comprehensive, well-researched book on perimenopause. Shonali shares anecdotes of her own experiences, while Nozer talks to us through case studies of patients. What is particularly uplifting is the message that this stage should be regarded as a period of transformation that women can and should emerge out of with energy, purpose and optimism. There are many books about menopause but, I say this as an accredited menopause specialist, if there is one that you must definitely choose, go for this and you will indeed find your balance'—Dr Azmy Birdi, menopause specialist and menopause special skills trainer

FINDING *Your* BALANCE

Your 360° Guide to
Perimenopause *and* Beyond

DR NOZER SHERIAR
SHONALI SABHERWAL

EBURY
PRESS

An imprint of Penguin Random House

EBURY PRESS

USA | Canada | UK | Ireland | Australia
New Zealand | India | South Africa | China

Ebury Press is part of the Penguin Random House group of companies
whose addresses can be found at global.penguinrandomhouse.com

Published by Penguin Random House India Pvt. Ltd
4th Floor, Capital Tower 1, MG Road,
Gurugram 122 002, Haryana, India

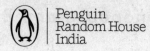

Penguin
Random House
India

First published in Ebury Press by Penguin Random House India 2022

ISBN 9780143441786

Typeset in Sabon by Manipal Technologies Limited, Manipal
Printed at Replika Press Pvt. Ltd, India

www.penguin.co.in

MIX
Paper from
responsible sources
FSC® C016779

This book is dedicated to our mothers, Dr Soonu Sheriar and Mrs Rajkumari Sabherwal, strong, sensitive and beautiful women. They inspired us, influenced us, supported us and made us what we are today.

Contents

Part Two
Deconstructing Clinical Situations and
Understanding Treatment Options

Part Three

Part Four
Guidance from Experts

The Four Heavenly Fountains

Laugh, I tell you
And you will turn back the hands of time.

Smile, I tell you
And you will reflect the face of the divine.

Sing, I tell you
And all the angels will sing with you!

Cry, I tell you
And the reflections found in your pool of tears—
Will remind you of the lessons of today and yesterday
To guide you through the fears of tomorrow.
                                            —Suzy Kassem

Foreword

Age Graciously. Age Well.

The trick is to age honestly and gracefully and make it look great so that everyone looks forward to it.

—Emma Thompson

I have always lived in the moment and looked forward to a beautiful tomorrow. In my life's journey, I have transitioned very easily from one phase to another. This, I contribute to my classical dance practice and performances, which instilled in me a great deal of discipline and commitment for the art and helped me develop simple food habits and an uncomplicated lifestyle. Being an early riser, I have always been able to dedicate a good amount of time to my morning routine. Coming from a highly disciplined family background, I have always been a family person and never indulged in consuming foods and drinks that I considered unhealthy.

I am a part of the film industry in which looking young, looking beautiful and living a larger-than-life kind of a lifestyle is the mantra. Just one look around our present world will tell the story of how everyone is shying away from age. There are a number of remedies now in the market to make a woman look twenty years younger.

Personally, I feel one should never place barriers for oneself at any stage of life. Instead, we must accept age gracefully. We ought to look at menopause, too, as just another stage in our lives, like puberty, pregnancy or ageing. If we accept this as the truth about our lives, everything else becomes a smooth experience.

I never felt pressured by the demands that the film industry puts on an actress. Hence, I worked as per my terms. Ageing for me became just another part of my life process. I accepted this process as my reality and so, it was easy for me to age gracefully. The result was that I started getting roles that suited my personality.

We women are always trying to defy age, look younger and be slimmer. How about focusing on just feeling good from the inside? This is what I have always striven towards. As a woman, I play many roles, and I try my best to do justice to all of them—whether as a daughter, a mother, a wife, a sister, a friend, a mother-in-law, an employer to a large staff, a grandmother and now a member of Parliament. While I wear many hats at any given time, just like all you women out there, I try to keep grounded with the tools I have used to stay healthy through the different phases of my life and accept my age. I can give you no better advice other than saying, keep it uncomplicated. I have never compromised on being healthy in mind and body. I have one other intrinsic trait, and that is that I am extremely self-reliant. As far as possible, I like to do things myself and depend less on others for anything.

The coming together of these two strong personalities in their respective fields, Dr Nozer Sheriar and Shonali Sabherwal, to give you the right framework to breeze through situations you might face in this phase of your life, is a blessing. When Shonali came to me to explain her book and how she and Dr Nozer wanted the book to be a go-to for everything that a woman goes through in the various stages of her midlife, I was happy to be a part of it, to help spread the principles of what a woman could potentially face and what tools she must use to navigate through the pre- and post-menopausal years, both medically and holistically.

For all of you out there, know this—it can be as hard or as easy to go through life as you make it. It just requires the right attitude, a very committed lifestyle, good food habits and the help of medical advances when needed.

Wishing you all a positive, youthful and a graceful life.

Hema Malini,
Member of Parliament, Lok Sabha,
Actress, dancer, director, producer, humanitarian

Book Outline

'You can't postpone the inevitable. The whole thing
about women is that they change. Men, poor old things
seem to go on in their same groove for their whole lives.'
— Germaine Greer

This book is written to address the perimenopause with a
holistic focus on dietary, lifestyle and therapeutic solutions.
It does this by following women's physical and emotional
journey as they prepare for, go through and finally spend
their lives after menopause.

With the modern woman spending a significant
part of her life being menopausal, she needs to recognize
and understand that this life-cycle transition is greatly
influenced by many factors which include hormonal
changes, food habits, physical activity and emotional
situation. These influences then translate into a variety of
clinical presentations and manifestations, which positively

or negatively impact general and reproductive health before, during or after menopause.

The contemporary woman is also faced with new and unique challenges in her everyday life. The book discusses how these stresses affect perimenopause and seeks to present the impact of lifestyle and environmental stressors. It also seeks to introduce women to their own hormones and help them recognize the reality and consequences of menopause as a hormone-deficiency state. The medical aspects of the book outline each hormone—why they are needed, their functions and the results of lack or excess that would lead to perimenopausal disturbances.

The content also focuses on the role of lifestyle—right diet, food triggers and exercise—that create a positive space for hormones to thrive in menopause and addresses aspects of menopause that impact ageing, bones, sexuality, the body and the mind and the association of hormones with general health and cancers. Using this book as guide we hope that women preparing for or living in the perimenopause stage will be able to draw individualized benefits as they negotiate the life-changing situations they will inevitably face.

Read the book to suit your personality. Devour it by reading it from cover to cover or savour it by nibbling at the edges. If you are impatient and looking for specifics, go straight to the relevant chapter or then use it as a reference volume to go back to time and again.

The book is written to be at once conversational and clinical, philosophical and medical, light and heavy. In fact, it is whatever you want it to be, so make it yours.

Introduction

Perimenopause: Insights and Understanding

Shonali Sabherwal: Personal Insights

This book comes at a perfect time in my life, as I sit at the brink of my menopause. I am in what they call perimenopause, the time in a woman's life shortly before her period stops, called the menopause, and I can see my body go through changes and my brain circuitry firing in different directions. I have no control, except towards my own attitude to this situation and the foundation which I have put in place. Years of healthy eating, regular exercise and meditation are strong stilts for going through my menopause.

As the world would say, I am in midlife and there is much more happening here than just my hormones going out of whack. The average age of women going through menopause is between forty-eight and fifty-five years, while in India that figure has been put at between forty-six and forty-eight years.* Even though the term 'midlife' has been used to describe this phase, I don't feel it one bit. I still feel twenty, running the streets of my campus in America, trying to catch my lecture, with my hair blowing in the wind and a spring in my step. I am under no illusion that I look like I am twenty, but I certainly don't feel it inside my head or my body, and most women at this point will say the same thing. We certainly look a lot younger than our mothers did at our age. You must have heard the phrase that the forties are the new thirties—well, that's just it. In a nutshell, I am declaring it right here and now, that women in their forties, fifties and sixties can no longer be considered women in midlife.

As I move through my life, I can see most of my friends and clients around me going through their perimenopause. Their complaints range from gaining weight despite being on diets and watching their food, feeling blue inexplicably, they say they are ratty and bark back at their spouse and kids. (On another note, after listening to them, I think if someone were to start a business to establish a support group for men whose women were going through menopause, they would do very well). They all begin to doubt themselves because most of them are simultaneously going through the empty-nest syndrome, settled in their marriages with no children between them any longer or, in today's scenario, there are a lot of women who are divorced, so there is this feeling of being 'alone'. They find themselves at a juncture in their life where they do not know how to chart a new road for themselves, and life suddenly becomes very daunting. Now, as I mentioned earlier, it is a matter of attitude, but it is

---

* Emedicine.com

also a matter of understanding the physical symptoms of where we women stand. Most of these women have turned life around on its head and gone raging into their fifties, having accepted what they are going through and forging new paths, careers, and lives.

Preparation for menopause begins very early, in the years post getting your period. Your lifestyle, diet and emotional factors set you up in the ageing process towards a tough or an easy menopause. I hope this book will be read by young women, early in life, as a preventive strategy for menopause.

One of the greatest gifts a doctor and healthcare practitioner can give their women patients is to prepare them to be healthy, content and happy perimenopausal women. This book is a labour of love with my gynaecologist and friend Dr Nozer Sheriar.

Nozer Sheriar: Professional Understanding

She was in her mid-sixties with two liver transplants. Fifteen years after menopause she was still symptomatic and on hormone therapy with estrogen patches, the preferred modality for her since, delivered through the skin, the hormone safely bypassed her precious liver. Every attempt to stop therapy had a recurrence of menopausal symptoms, so this brave and strong woman made an informed choice to continue estrogen therapy well beyond the notional upper limit of five years. This makes this case atypical and a complete outlier. Maybe this is not the case to start this book with, but it highlights for me the fact that every woman is different and unique with varied presentations, needs and solutions.

While every woman has her own perimenopausal story, as a gynaecologist and a doctor who cares for women, I have a thousand such stories. Each one is about the same inevitable change in a woman's life and yet completely different. Women lead many sequential hormonal lives—childhood, adolescence, childbearing years, pre-menopause and a long life after menopause. Each of these is fascinating but for me none more so than the subject of this book—the perimenopause.

While menopause has always been an integral part of women's lives, it is only in the last fifty years that society and the medical profession have developed the capacity to give it the importance it deserves. With women now living longer than at any time in human history, a third of their lives will be spent in perimenopause. They also live in a time when the physiological and hormonal changes related to menopause have been demystified and we now have the capacity, tools and treatments to prevent, protect against and manage associated problems.

Hormone treatment of menopause started in the sixties when gynaecologist Robert Wilson published his bestselling book *Feminine Forever* in 1966. He maintained that menopause was an estrogen-deficiency disease that should be treated with estrogen-replacement therapy to prevent, what he crudely and obnoxiously termed as the inevitable living decay. The book coincided with the rise of the feminist movement; while some embraced the use of estrogens as a boon for ageing women, others resisted and steadfastly refused to accept the notion that female ageing was pathological. In 1975, there was a backlash with studies linking the use of high-dose synthetic estrogens with uterine cancer, challenging the wisdom of routine hormone therapy and shifting the tenor of feminist discussion.

Since then, a rational thought process evolved with the consensus that menopause is a natural, physiological, hormone-deficiency state. For most women, its symptoms are mild and easily tolerated, requiring reassurance and understanding, a focus on self-care and protection and sensible dietary, exercise and lifestyle change. For those whose menopausal symptoms were distressing, a medical treatment option, mainly centred on hormone-replacement therapy using low-dose natural estrogens, was clearly defined.

Then, in 2002, the Women's Health Initiative (WHI), created panic by reporting that hormone therapy had more detrimental, than beneficial, effects. With that, HRT use dropped, since the negative results received wide and exaggerated media coverage, creating panic among both users and doctors. Fortunately, in the following years a re-analysis of the trial showed that the WHI results were skewed and not representative for most women and that the use of indicated HRT in younger and early post-menopausal women had beneficial effects. This knee-jerk reaction to what was perceived as negative news denied a large number of women justifiable medical care and demonstrated to me that the medical management of menopause, a crossroad in every woman's life, will always be at risk of opinion and conjecture, judgement and overreaction. Hence this book and my partnership with Shonali, an acclaimed macrobiotic nutritionist, a lifestyle guide, a much-published author and a dear friend. There exist many contemporary medical guidelines on menopause care based on latest evidence and in this book, we refer to them. Of these, the International Menopause Society and the Indian Menopause Society recommendations on women's midlife health and menopause hormone therapy are the ones we have referred to the most.

This book has at its heart a concern for the quality of life for women. It is arranged so as to walk with you through your perimenopausal journey, to be your guide to address and offer solutions for your complaints and to be a go-to resource for questions that you, dear readers, may have. Ladies, read it for yourself; men, read it for your partner. Read it for your present and for your future.

Part One

Preparing Yourself to
Navigate the Perimenopause

'All things are ready, if our mind be so.'

—William Shakespeare

1

Reaching Midlife: Ushering in Something New

'A lot of people resist transition and therefore never allow themselves to enjoy who they are. Embrace the change, no matter what it is; once you do, you can learn about the new world you're in and take advantage of it.'

—Nikki Giovanni

Nozer Sheriar: Defining Your Midlife

How do you know whether you have reached your midlife or your perimenopause? You are said to have reached your natural menopause when you have no periods for twelve months with the absence of any medical problems. This occurs when you have used up all or almost all the egg (oocyte) containing follicles in your ovary, resulting in a dramatic fall in estrogen levels, medically described as hypoestrogenism.

3

The transition process and the time immediately before and after menopause is referred to as the **perimenopause** or the **climacteric**. Incidentally, the word climacteric is derived from a Greek word meaning *rung of a ladder,* an elegant statement of a woman's stepping upwards as she reaches midlife. This transition begins an average of four years before the final menstrual period and includes a number of natural changes that may affect a woman's quality of life. It is characterized by irregular menstrual cycles and marked hormonal fluctuations.

There are three terms we need to define so that you can identify the stages that women go through during the climacteric.

First, there is the **pre-menopause**. This term is used to describe the early years of the climacteric, generally after forty years. It has been divided into an early phase which is variable and a late phase of one to three years.

Second, there is the **menopause**. This is a definitive event that has a date and is the final menstrual period in a woman's life. It is a biological landmark in a woman's life that marks the end of her natural reproductive life. Menopause is generally confirmed retrospectively when there are no periods for twelve consecutive months after the last period.

Third, there is the **post-menopause**. This is the time after menopause has occurred, starting when you have not had a period for twelve consecutive months. This too has an early phase and a late phase.

The overarching **perimenopause** is the stage lasting for several years on either side of the last menstrual period. It is the menopause transition and is characterized by irregular menstrual cycles, endocrine changes and symptoms such as hot flushes that may affect a woman's quality of life.

The biology and symptomatology of menopause are blurred due to their relationship to the underlying ageing process. To better understand the transition from reproductive years through menopause, we share with you a staging system that was developed for the medical care of perimenopause. This is now considered to be the gold standard for classifying stages in your reproductive ageing. It is called the STRAW (Stages of Reproductive Ageing Workshop) staging system. It divides women's lives into phases using menstrual changes, hormonal changes and ultrasound findings. Refer to the chart in Figure 1 to determine where you stand based upon your history and other parameters.

Figure 1: The STRAW +10 staging system for reproductive ageing

Phase	Reproduction				Transition		Post menopause			
Stage	-5	-4	-3b	-3a	-2	-1	+1a	+1b	+1c	+2
Duration	Early	Peak	Late		Perimenopause			Early		Late
	Variable				Variable	1-3 years	2 years	3-6 years		Lifelong
Principal menstrual criteria										
Menses	Variable to regular	Regular	Regular	Subtle changes in flow length	Variable with 7 day differences	Intervals with no periods over 60 days	No periods			
Supportive endocrine criteria										
FSH AMH			Low Low	Variable Low	↑Variable Low	↑ >25 IU/L Low	↑ Variable Low	Stabilizes Very low		
AFC			Low	Low	Low	Low	Very low	Very low		
Descriptive symptomatic criteria										
Symptoms							Vasomotor likely			Urogenital likely

Menarche
First period

Menopause
Last period

Shonali Sabherwal: Ushering in Something New

I, for one, find myself ushering in a new phase in my life. This phase is forcing me to ask questions about where I am and where I'd like to be. I am uncovering a wisdom that has been there for ages and which I am just pulling out from the hidden recesses of my mind and experiences. I feel I have become young all over again and can live my life all over, like I did in my twenties. This stage has forced me to examine myself under a microscope, even as a person. I have worked out my past issues, I know myself better than I ever did, I am comfortable in my own skin, I have worked hard enough to earn the place and space I am in, I know a lot about my subject so no one can bullshit me, I have survived being single and a woman and most of all I am happy being exactly where I am and where I am supposed to be.

I feel our hormones are a gift at this time, as they compel us to look at our own lives in the eye and ask ourselves whether we need to change some stuff that's not right. So, if any of you who are reading this are feeling the same way, then let's use this time to truly own the second half of our lives. Let's not just react to it but be present and appreciate the mysteries it brings.

A lot of my mom's menopause had to do with her attitude in life towards stuff she went through in general. She marched to her own drum in her approach to society, the world and the universe at large. She has been a tough nut, as most would say, very strong, extremely practical and very comfortable with who she is. When I asked her whether she remembers when she went through menopause and whether she went through a tough perimenopause, her answer was: 'Not at all. One day I woke up and my period was gone and never came back after that.'

There was no build up, no drama; she even said, 'I don't know why women make such a fuss nowadays before they reach menopause.' While this is the story of my mother, my ex-mother-in-law had quite a different story. She really suffered. I remember her saying that she would go through three packets of sanitary pads in a day because of the heavy bleeding and the passing of clots. She complained of severe pain and was irritable and moody as well.

Dr Raveendran, my Ayurvedic doctor and friend, says, 'do not label an illness, as it becomes you.' I can extend that analogy to menopause. Do not keep labelling it as 'I am going through menopause', as it becomes you. I see most women doing this today; our mothers never did so. They considered menopause as a normal bodily adjustment, just like getting a period. Menopause should be simply viewed as a change in a woman's biological life, moving away from her younger, childbearing years to a period of power, achievement and having arrived, instead of being viewed as a period of symptoms, that might or might not come about.

During this period, my dear, you are likely to experience an urge for freedom and spontaneity. Under all that subliminal negative energy, you have positive energy, which is genius energy to create new things and move away from the mundane, daily stuff, a consciousness that does not define you. You are on the brink of a transformation. Believe me when I say your mental state will transcend to something bigger and brighter. You will move into new ways of thinking and being, which may need you to alter your lifestyle. There may be changes in store for you that have been waiting for the right moment to come in; new ways of being that when exercised, will change you.

You will go through pain. You can't make gold until it is smelted through fire. It may leave you vulnerable for a while, you may feel exposed, but something will propel you in new directions. Please acknowledge the wisdom that comes to you through this phase, because you will come out of it stronger. This is a time to dissolve old habits and structures and move towards the new.

The story of La Loba*

There is a story about La Loba, the wolf woman, who lives among the granite slopes in Tarahumara Indian territory. She is called by many names—La Loba, the wolf woman, Huesera, the bone woman and La Trapera, the gatherer. Her sole work is collecting bones. She is known to collect and preserve that which is in danger of being lost to the world.

She sifts through the mountains and riverbeds, looking for wolf bones. When she has assembled an entire skeleton, when the last bone is in place and the beautiful white sculpture of the creature is laid out before her, she sits by the fire and sings. She stands over the creature, raises her arms over it and sings out. That is when the bones of the ribcage and the leg bones of the wolf begin to flesh out and the creature becomes furred. She sings some more and more of the creature comes into being, its tail curling upward, shaggy and strong. As she continues to sing, the wolf creature begins to breathe. And then La Loba sings so deeply that the floor of the desert shakes and as she sings, the wolf opens its eyes, leaps forward and bounds away down the canyon.

Somewhere in its running, the wolf is suddenly transformed into a laughing woman who runs free towards the horizon. It is said that if you wander the desert near

---

* Clarissa Pinkola Estés, *Women Who Run With the Wolves*, Ballantine Books, 1992, pp. 12, 25–30.

sundown and if you are lucky, La Loba may take a liking to you and show you something of her soul.

We all begin as a bundle of bones lost somewhere in the desert, a dismantled skeleton lying under the sand. It is our work to recover the parts, a painstaking process best done when the shadows are just right, for it takes much looking. La Loba indicates what we are to look for—the indestructible life force.

A healthy woman is much like a wolf, robust and chock-full of a strong life force, life-giving, loyal and territorial. Separation from her primal nature causes a woman's personality to become thin, ghostly and spectral. We are not meant to be puny and unable to leap up, to chase, to birth, to create life. When women's lives are in stasis, it is time for the wildish, self-confident, self-reliant woman of awareness to emerge.

For me, the story of La Loba is what we women should be doing—gathering up our bones and resurrecting ourselves to prepare for a new phase in our lives. Great power comes when we accept our situation for what it is, hold ourselves accountable for where we are and take complete responsibility for our problems. With this, the attitude of why-me ceases and the attitude of why-not-me comes in. While there is more comfort in hanging on to the old patterns in our lives, it is a time of transformation, so why not allow this new energy to take us over? To face a marriage that has become difficult, go through a divorce, have your children leave home or seem like they do not need you any more, break up a long-standing relationship, these are all problems with gifts.

Christiane Northrup, an obstetrician and gynaecologist, says:

Menopause may not feel like a rescue at the time, but the clarity of vision and increasing intolerance for injustice, inequity and lack of fulfilment that accompany perimenopausal changes are a gift. Our hormones are giving us an opportunity to see, once and for all, what we need to change in order to live honestly, fully, joyfully, and healthfully in the second half of our lives. This is the time when many women stop doing what I call 'stuffing'—stifling their own needs in order to tend to everyone else's.[*]

* Christiane Northrup, *The Wisdom of Menopause: Creating Physical and Emotional Health During the Change*, Bantam, 2012, p. 19.

2

Hormone Primer: A Closer Look at Hormones

'The maturing of a woman who has continued to grow is a beautiful thing to behold.'

—Naomi Wolf

If we were to explain hormones to you in one sentence, they are like your body's lines of communication—phone calls, text messages, WhatsApp or Emails. They travel from one part of the body to the other and are responsible for keeping your physical and mental balance. Like all channels of communication that operate in a virtual space, they have the ability to enter every cell of your body and also your brain.

Let's Get Closer to Your Hormones

To understand the perimenopause, you have to understand your hormones, so we present herewith a brief, albeit slightly complicated, lesson in human physiology.

Your reproductive hormones belong to a chemical class called steroids. The two main classes of sex steroids or sex hormones are estrogens and androgens, of which the most important human derivatives are estradiol and testosterone respectively. Progestogens are considered the third class of sex steroids, with progesterone being the most important.

In general, estrogens and progestogens are considered 'female sex hormones' and androgens are considered 'male sex hormones', although all of them are present in both sexes in different levels and concentrations. These hormones affect all parts of the body: the brain, the circulation system, the bones, the digestive system, the liver, the reproductive organs and also your immune system.

Sex steroids include all the following hormones:

- **Estrogens**
  - 2-Hydroxyestrone → **Estrone**
  - 2-Hydroxyestradiol → **Estradiol** → **Estriol**
- **Progestogens**
  - Pregnenolone → **Progesterone**
  - 17α-Hydroxypregnenolone →
    17α-Hydroxyprogesterone
- **Androgens**
  - Dehydroepiandrosterone → Androstenedione
  - Androstenediol → **Testosterone** →
    Dihydrotestosterone

All sex hormones are derived from cholesterol. They are made by the ovaries or the testes, the adrenal glands or by the conversion from other sex steroids in the fat or the liver. From a common source, their production is interlinked, and they have the ability to be made from one another, depending upon the needs of the body. There is a flow or cascade (Figure 2) from cholesterol through progestogens and androgens to estrogens, so if one of the links is compromised or missing, this could have a domino effect.

Figure 2: Interrelated production of sex steroid hormones

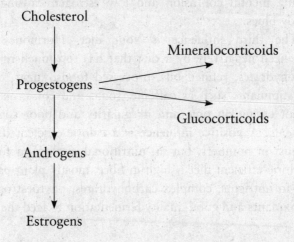

Factors Affecting Hormonal Balance

A number of factors determine whether your hormones are going to stay in balance or be disturbed.

The first influence is the balance of your vitamins, minerals and enzymes. You need vitamins and minerals as cofactors to transform one hormone into another.

Enzymes are large molecules continuously created from our chromosomes. They act as catalysts to bring about specific biochemical reactions, including hormone production.

The second influence is stress. This can play havoc with hormones and vice versa, a Catch-22 situation you can get caught in. With stress, the adrenal glands secrete more cortisol. When cortisol and adrenaline are released, they raise your cholesterol level, which is the stuff that steroid hormones are made of. Thus, stress feeds the imbalance of hormones and then hormones feed off the stress. Estrogen can fire up the brain, with estrogen dominance and excess causing mental confusion and low estrogen causing the moody blues.

The third influence is your diet. Hormones are influenced negatively by a diet that has too much refined carbohydrates, refined oils, processed foods, sugar, dairy and stimulants such as caffeine, sodas and colas, as also by not eating on time and irregularity and poor spacing of meals. A positive influence is a calorie-efficient diet— not just in numbers, but in 'nutritional quality' of foods. A calorie-efficient diet is high in fibre, mostly plant-based, high in nutrients, complex carbohydrates, phytoestrogens, antioxidants and good quality fermentation to feed the gut.

The Cholesterol Connection in the Perimenopause

Shonali's cholesterol went up a couple of months ago. She immediately realized that it was the perimenopause phase with its fluctuating progesterone and estrogen levels that was the cause and not liquid fat like oil or other forms of fat that she had consumed with food. A lot of perimenopausal women would think they should cut back the fat in their diets, but that is not the solution.

When sugars and fats are broken down in the liver, cholesterol is a by-product. During this phase, a lot of women say their sugar cravings go up, but it is quite the opposite. It is a sedentary lifestyle and a bad diet that drives the craving for more sugars, subsequently leading to higher cholesterol levels.

A zero-fat diet is a bad idea, since the building block for all hormones is cholesterol. While our body makes cholesterol from the foods we eat, a fourth comes from foods that actually have cholesterol. If these foods are eliminated, you may suffer from a hormonal imbalance.

Knowing Your Endocrine System

Your endocrine system is a network of glands in your body that make hormones, which are responsible for almost every cell, organ and function in your body. Some glands such as the pituitary direct the work of other glands, while others such as the ovaries, testes and adrenals deliver the actual hormones. Some glands such as the thyroid, parathyroid and pancreas have specialized functions. It is quite a democratic system in which all the glands communicate with each other, giving feedback messages to optimize function.

Figure 3: The components of the endocrine network

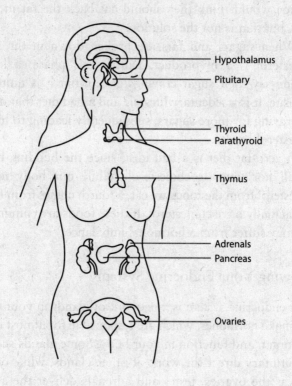

- Hypothalamus
- Pituitary
- Thyroid
- Parathyroid
- Thymus
- Adrenals
- Pancreas
- Ovaries

The Key Hormones

We Start with Estrogen

Shonali's niece, Zara, is all of eleven years old, 5 feet 6 inches tall, and has already had her first period. The fact that she has hit puberty indicates that estrogen has surged in her system. This will stop her long bones from developing any further, which means she may not increase in height. Estrogen stimulates cell growth. Its job is to give the female body the signal to build the uterine lining in the first part of the menstrual cycle and is a part of the hormonal signal that stimulates the maturation of an egg-containing follicle in the ovary. Think of estrogen in your body as a dynamic entity, changing as life moves along.

At this juncture, understanding estrogen is important in your quest for hormonal balance. Achieving the right balance of estrogen is much like striving to maintain your weight—done well by those women who are consistent with the right diet and exercise to keep themselves healthy; it is a long process that begins much before a woman hits perimenopause.

The word estrogen describes compounds with estrogenic properties and is actually not the name of a specific hormone. They range from human estrogens, animal estrogens, synthetic estrogens and phytoestrogens to xenoestrogens. The three main human estrogens are estradiol, estrone and estriol. Produced in the ovaries, the adrenal glands and in small quantities in body fat, estrogen is responsible for the development and maintenance of female sexual traits like breasts and also the uterine lining. Any excess or deficiency will create chaos within the body.

Estradiol (E2 as indicated on blood tests) is the major female sex hormone that is produced within the follicles of the ovaries, the adrenals, the fat tissue, the liver, the breasts and the brain. It is involved in the regulation of menstrual cycles and is responsible for secondary sexual characteristics such as the widening of the hips and a female-associated pattern of fat and hair distribution. It is responsible for the development of the breasts, uterus and vagina and also acts on the bone, the fat, the skin, the liver and the brain. After menopause, the production of estrogens by the ovaries stops and estradiol levels decrease to very low levels.

Estrone (E1 as indicated on your blood tests) is a weak estrogen and a minor female sex hormone. Estrone is mainly secreted from the ovaries, although it can also be formed from adrenal androgens in fat tissue. It is an important hormone for women who have gone through menopause as it becomes their major source of estrogen. An important factor to consider is a well-functioning liver, as most of the estrone is converted in the liver into estradiol after menopause.

Estriol (E3 as indicated on your blood test) is also a weak estrogen and a minor female sex hormone. While estriol is synthesized in very high quantities by the placenta during pregnancy, its levels in women who are not pregnant are almost undetectable. This weak estrogen is occasionally used as a medication for menopausal symptoms.

Enter Progesterone

During the reproductive years, the follicle-stimulating hormone (FSH) and the luteinizing hormone (LH) are produced by the pituitary gland placed just below the brain. FSH induces the growth and maturation of a new egg and its release from its ovarian follicle every month. As the follicle develops, it produces estrogen throughout and progesterone in the second half of the cycle. Both are responsible for the thickening of the uterus lining every month before you get your menstrual cycle. Progesterone levels increase in the second half of the menstrual cycle, after the release of an egg.

Progesterone is associated with fertility and pregnancy. It is secreted by the ovaries in a woman's menstruating life. The corpus luteum is a temporary endocrine structure that develops from the empty follicle after ovulation. It produces estrogen and progesterone, maintaining optimum conditions for implantation if the egg is fertilized. Once pregnancy occurs, the corpus luteum persists and plays an important role through the first trimester. Progesterone is made from the sterol pregnenolone, which in turn is derived from cholesterol.

Progesterone, if not utilized, passes through the liver and is then excreted. As mentioned earlier, it is a major precursor for estrogen and testosterone. It rises after ovulation, when it is significantly higher in the body and then drops when there is no fertilization of the egg. This fall in progesterone is when you shed your uterine lining and get your period.

In macrobiotics, we base our understanding of everything upon the principle of *chi,* or *ki* and prana in Indian terminology. This is described as the universal life force around us, which splits into *yin* (female/expansive energy) and *yang* (male/contractive energy). These two forces are complimentary yet antagonistic. The same analogy can be applied to estrogen and progesterone. Progesterone functions on the basis of estrogen and balances many of its effects.

Natural progesterone has gained popularity in recent years and is now used to control symptoms of premenstrual-like syndrome and perimenopause. It is given in small doses to balance estrogen.

It is fascinating to know what estrogen and progesterone do for you. A closer look makes it obvious that estrogen and progesterone are closely linked, with different yet complementary effects.

Estrogen Effects	Progesterone Effects
Creates proliferative endometrium	Maintains secretory endometrium
Breast-cell stimulation	Protects against fibrocystic breasts
Increased body fat and weight gain	Helps use fat for energy
Salt and fluid retention	Natural diuretic
Depression, anxiety and headaches	Natural antidepressant calms anxiety
Cyclical migraines	
Poor sleep patterns	Promotes normal sleep patterns
Interferes with thyroid function	Facilitates thyroid hormones
Impairs blood-sugar control	Helps normalize blood-sugar levels
Increased risk of blood clots	Normalizes blood clotting
Little or no libido effect	Helps restore normal libido
Loss of zinc and retention of copper	Normalizes zinc and copper levels
Reduced oxygen levels in all cells	Restores proper levels of oxygen in the cell
Related to endometrial cancer	Prevents endometrial cancer
Increased risk of breast cancer	Prevents breast cancer
Slows bone loss	Stimulates new bone formation
Reduces vascular tone	Improves vascular tone
Triggers autoimmune disease	Prevents autoimmune disease

Androgens in Women

Now that we've looked at the two major female-dominant hormones and the interplay between them, let us discuss androgens. When you think of androgens, you think of everything male. But you would be surprised to know that women produce androgens as well. These include androstenedione, testosterone, dihydrotestosterone (DHT) and dehydroepiandrosterone (DHEA). Referred to as the male hormones, they produce masculine effects like growth of facial hair and other male traits. Androgens act as mediators in the body's production of estrogen. In women, they are equally secreted by the ovaries and the adrenal glands and have a marginal, although important, effect on her wellbeing.

Testosterone is the primary male sex hormone and an anabolic steroid. It is secreted by the testes in males and the ovaries in females with contribution from the adrenal glands in both. In adult men, levels of testosterone are eight times higher than women, although women seem to be more sensitive to the hormone. Women's testosterone levels decline significantly as they approach menopause and continue to do so post-menopause. The ovaries, however, continue to produce testosterone in small amounts even after menopause.

One of the most important functions of testosterone is to maintain libido in women. One of the reasons why women experience a loss of sexual desire in the perimenopause is a declining testosterone. A deficiency of testosterone may also cause lack of energy, vaginal dryness, loss of sex drive and memory loss. Besides this, it is the interplay of androgens that determines skin health in women.

Dehydroepiandrosterone (DHEA as indicated on blood tests) is made in the adrenal glands. Both estrogen and testosterone are made from DHEA. Apart from being a precursor for the formation of other hormones, it also contributes to keeping one's immunity up. When Shonali's DHEA levels had dropped considerably, she found she was constantly exhausted and stressed out, suggesting that her adrenals were in push mode. DHEA, when low, could be a precursor to autoimmune disease, cancer, diabetes and even heart issues. It has been known to help with the ageing process and supplementation helps with hair health, osteoporosis and longevity. A large amount of DHEA is bound and ready to be accessed when required. DHEA has been used to boost energy and wellness, to deal with stress and to help with libido.

Androstenedione is also made in the adrenals and ovaries and is a precursor to estrogen and testosterone. In the perimenopause, it converts to estrogen in the fat cells. Androstenedione increases muscle mass and is hence popular among weightlifters and athletes. It also helps with protecting bones by converting to estradiol, which then slows down bone loss. The US Food and Drug Administration (FDA) advises against the use of androstenedione as a supplement to enhance these effects. Being an androgen, it may affect development of facial hair and deepening of the voice in women.

Other Important Hormones

Thyroid Hormones

The thyroid gland is a butterfly-shaped endocrine gland that lies in the front of the neck. It secretes two hormones, thyroxine (T4) and triiodothyronine (T3). The T4 is converted to T3 in your cells and body tissues. The T3 derived from T4 directly influences metabolism, regulating the speed with which your cells work and how your body uses energy. If you have too much of the thyroid hormones, the body cells work faster and you will develop hyperthyroidism (overactive thyroid) with symptoms of unintentional weight loss, even when your appetite and food intake remain the same or increase; other symptoms include rapid heartbeat, palpitations, increased appetite, nervousness, anxiety and irritability. If, on the other hand, too little of the thyroid hormones are produced, you develop hypothyroidism (underactive thyroid) with symptoms of fatigue, increased sensitivity to cold, constipation, dry skin, weight gain, puffy face and muscle weakness.

Thyroid-Stimulating Hormone (TSH) is the hormone secreted by the pituitary gland that controls thyroid function and is used to assess thyroid health or dysfunction. When thyroid levels in your body are low, the pituitary gland makes more TSH. When thyroid levels are high, the pituitary gland makes less TSH. So TSH levels that are high or low can indicate your thyroid is not working correctly.

Cortisol

Cortisol is the body's main stress hormone. The adrenal glands that sit on top of the kidneys make cortisol. It works with the brain to influence your moods and influences your response to stress and fear. The hypothalamus and pituitary gland—both located in your brain—can sense if your blood contains the right amounts of cortisol. When you encounter a perceived threat, the hypothalamus sets off an alarm system in your body. This prompts the adrenals to release adrenaline and cortisol. If the levels are too low, then the brain adjusts the amount of hormones it makes accordingly. The adrenal glands also pick this up and adjust cortisol levels. Cortisol receptors, which are in most cells in the body, receive and use this hormone in different ways— to influence digestive function, reproductive function and many growth processes. If the adrenals are under constant pressure and the cortisol levels go out of whack, it can interfere with many of your body's functions.

Cortisol manages how your body will use carbohydrates, manages blood-sugar levels, helps keep inflammation under check, controls your sleep cycles, regulates blood pressure, boosts energy levels, affects the immune-system response and brings the body back into balance. Long-term stress will disrupt normal cortisol levels and put you at a risk for anxiety, thyroid issues, depression, weight gain, muscle ache, sleep issues, digestive problems, heart disease and memory issues.

Insulin

Insulin helps keep the body's blood sugar levels and metabolism under check. It also helps turn the food you eat into energy. The pancreas make insulin and releases it into the bloodstream. After a meal, the intestines break down the carbohydrates from the food into glucose, which then enters the bloodstream, increasing the blood-sugar levels. The body makes and releases insulin in a feedback loop based on your blood-sugar levels. The more the blood-sugar levels increase, the more the insulin secreted by the pancreas. As soon as the sugar moves into the cells, the blood-sugar levels go back to normal. Low blood sugar prompts the pancreas to release glucagon. Both insulin and glucagon alternate their release through the day to keep blood-sugar levels in balance.

If you rely on a refined carbohydrate diet, poor nutrition choices like a lot of sugar and sugary foods and have long gaps in between meals, this system gets dysfunctional and can lead to type-2 diabetes. Insulin insensitivity signifies the body's inability to have this hormone function normally. Insulin resistance refers to low insulin sensitivity. With insulin resistance, the cells do not absorb glucose, causing hypersecretion of insulin. This leads to weight gain and elevated blood-sugar levels.

3

Preparing for Perimenopause: Transcending Midlife Barriers

'Take care of your body. It's the only place you have to live.'

—Jim Rohn

I describe myself as an active and healthy someone, who has lived life very consciously from my twenties, pretty much the time one starts to be an adult and assume one's own responsibility. My friend's dad, Sunil, calls me 'Getz Aug Go Go' after American saxophonist Stan Getz's album. Why? because my nick name is Gogi and some call me 'Go Go', including my dad and Sunil. I think they call me this to basically say I'm always on the go. That's how I also view myself.

I've always had a flat stomach, never an iota of fat sticking out, no love handles or visceral fat around the belly. Yet, I have started noticing a dramatic change in the last year or so. No matter what I do, this stubborn fat doesn't budge. I watch my diet and my exercise routine is as intense as it has always been. Despite all of this, it's like my body is doing its own jig.

I have some friends who have gone through this phase, and I have heard horror stories from them. Frankly, even though I am in the perimenopause phase of my life, I am not suffering that much, except for the body sending me signals of not wanting to shed weight. Like I mentioned earlier, this is the result of cultivating an attitude of 'going with the flow', accepting this phase and 'letting go.'

Preparing for menopause should begin early on in a woman's life. We women know that we are going to go through a midlife change. By this time, we have dealt with marriages and divorces, relationships and children, job changes and instability and issues with the self. I think we can safely agree that we are, at this stage, less likely to make excuses for anything, accept responsibility and speak our truth. We now want to focus on our selves. At forty-two, I have dealt with all the issues I had. I have used my meditation practice and psychotherapy; I am done with dead-end relationships; I am happy with my bulky thighs; I know the lines on my face are there to stay; I have narrowed down my circle of friends to those that are going to be around me for life and made new ones who resonate with my energy. I speak my truth and don't make excuses for anything if I really believe in it. In short, I have come into my own and started preparing myself for what is to come. These are your best years, as your struggles on every level are now over. Please believe in this.

Shonali Sabherwal

Looking at Your Life under a Microscope

Our minds are increasingly conditioned with what Dr Google dishes out to us on any complaint, symptom or ailment. This has resulted in certain belief patterns about menopause—that what we go through is largely because of the havoc our hormones are playing in our bodies. We live a separate life in our minds from our bodies, imagining our hormones are not connected to our past, what we have been through and the stresses that life gives us.

The common thread we see in the menopause stories that we have heard from the many lives we have been exposed to is that the women who have an attitude of acceptance and have been resilient have had easier transitions into their menopause. In contrast, there are those women who take on life's stresses and let these fester in their minds, with a consequent impact on their bodies.

Paying close attention to how you react to situations in the mid-thirties, the decade before you go through perimenopause, and correcting belief patterns and attitudes is a good place to start. The build-up to a menopause is the time to take your health in your hands by re-examining how you eat, how you resolve emotional issues, letting go of people you cling to and clearing the unwanted clutter that surrounds your life. It is the time to put your life under a microscope and steer it in your chosen direction.

Christiane Northrup explains how the brain reacts and responds to menopause. She writes:

Like the rising heat on our bodies, our brains also become fired up! Sparked by hormonal changes that are typical during the menopausal transition, a switch goes on that signals changes in our temporal lobes, the brain region associated with enhanced intuition.[*]

How this ultimately affects us depends to a large degree on how willing we are to make the changes in our lives that our hormones are urging us to make over the ten years or so of perimenopause. She draws our attention to the body's inner wisdom and how to pay attention to the times in our lives when our body throws up signals.

- The first wake-up call is the pre-menstrual syndrome (PMS).

PMS is one way a woman's body nudges her each month to remind her of the growing backlog of unresolved issues accumulating within her. It is a reflection of hormonal fluctuation, and anything from unbalanced nutrition to unresolved relationships can contribute to disrupt the hormonal environment, wreaking physical and emotional havoc.

---

[*] Northrup, Christiane, *The Wisdom of Menopause: Creating Physical and Emotional Health During the Change*, Bantam Books, 2011, p. 38.

- The second wake-up call is post-partum depression.

If you have PMS, you are more likely to have post-partum depression in the first few weeks of giving birth. With a strong hormonal component, it may also signal emotional issues and relationships that need resolving, as do certain areas of a woman's life.

- The third wake-up call is seasonal affective disorder (SAD).

Described as more a phenomenon in the western world, this is a type of depression that is related to the marked change in seasons. It is connected to daylight getting shorter which in the West, in temperate climate zones, starts in Autumn and goes into Winter. SAD is when PMS symptoms intensify and get worse with the onset of winter and could lead to depression.

- The fourth wake-up call is the perimenopause.

The perimenopause is sometimes described as 'PMS times ten'. Stress has a lot to do with how perimenopause in your life will play out. Christiane Northrup observes that, '. . . an average woman, blessed with 480 menstrual periods and 40 seasonal cycles to bring her to the threshold of her menopause, gets about 500 progress reports.' To understand these reports, you need to ask yourself the following questions:

- How are my emotions?
- What's happening in my relationships and my career?

- Am I scheduling pleasure into my daily life or putting myself last?

You have approximately 500 opportunities to either resolve those issues positively or sweep them under the rug. At perimenopause, the process escalates. The earnest, straightforward inner self, which has tried for years to get your attention, makes one final, hormonally mediated attempt to get you to deal with your accumulated needs, wants and desires. This is likely to turn into a period of great emotional turmoil, as each woman struggles to make a new life, one that can accommodate her emerging self. Externally and internally, this period is a mirror image of adolescence, a time when bodies and brains go through major hormonal shifts that give us the energy to attempt to individuate and become the person we were meant to be.

For a woman, it is not her actual hormone levels, but a unique combination of hormones, brain chemistry and life situations that results in her symptoms.*

It is estimated that 27 per cent of women who experience agitation and depression during their periods and 36 per cent of women who are pre-menstrually depressed will be very sensitive to the hormonal changes that occur at menopause.

It is perimenopause, the fourth wakeup call that is important for us to focus on. The perimenopause phase in a woman's life is far more important and difficult to handle than menopause itself. While menopause is an event, the pre-menopause and perimenopause phases last for a long time. For most women, this transitional phase generally

---

* Ibid.

starts post thirty-five and gets pretty intense two years before the actual menopause.

You need to step back from your life and know where you are and what you can do about it, both medically and on the diet front. How you will handle your menopause is largely dependent on your diet and lifestyle and how you deal with stress and exhaustion.

How Do You Reach the Diagnosis of Menopause?

Menopause is diagnosed retrospectively. Menstrual irregularity is the only objective marker to define and establish the menopause transition. However, hormonal markers for diagnosis of menopause may be used when indicated. Levels of follicle-stimulating hormone (FSH) over 10 IU/L indicate declining ovarian function. FSH levels over 20 IU/L suggest ovarian insufficiency in the perimenopause with vasomotor symptoms (VMS), even if you are menstruating. An FSH level over 40 IU/L at least four weeks apart is a reliable marker for menopause or impending menopause and is associated with low estradiol levels. Anti-Mullerian hormone (AMH) becomes undetectable, and antral follicular count and ovarian volume decrease at menopause.

What Is the Average Age of Menopause in India?

The estimated mean age of menopause is forty-six years in India, which is lower than that of your Western counterparts. This earlier menopause predisposes Indian women to chronic health disorders a decade earlier, making perimenopausal care and this book on perimenopause solutions all the more important. From the available Indian data, the earlier age of menopause predisposes Indian women to osteoporotic fractures ten to twenty years earlier, type-2 diabetes mellitus a decade earlier and the breast-cancer peak before the age of fifty years.

What Is the Role of Accessory Hormones and Stress at Perimenopause

The purpose of the adrenals is to help the body cope with the onslaught of stress; they are also called 'glands of stress'. When your body faces a stressful condition, it will go into a 'fight or flight' mode causing the cortisol levels to increase. The adrenal and thyroid connection originates in the brain.

The adrenal glands' primary job is to produce just the right amount of stress hormones to help you to respond to all kinds of stress affecting you. Usually, a way to judge just how depleted you are is to see if you have the energy to get up and go in the mornings, called 'rising cortisol'.

The thyroid's main job is to produce just the right amount of thyroid hormones to tell your cells how fast they should burn energy and produce proteins. Think of the thyroid and adrenal glands as the gatekeepers of your endocrine system. They are continuously relaying information back and forth between the brain and the body.

You need just the right amount of cortisol for your thyroid to function optimally. Too much (from acute stress) or too little (as a result of continuous stress over time) can lead to problems. Imbalances along either axis that relays messages from the brain can result in either overactive or underactive adrenal glands, as well as an underactive thyroid. The thyroid receptors (which facilitate T3 action) can become less responsive. This may be one reason that symptoms of thyroid dysfunction can show up even when your thyroid lab tests appear 'within normal limits'.

Here's how this happens: Much of the medical literature looking at the effects of stress on the thyroid has focused on hyperthyroidism and a condition called Graves' disease. In general, Graves' is caused by an autoimmune response that prompts the thyroid to make too much thyroid hormone. This is known to occur after a sudden stressful life change in people with a specific genetic makeup. But much less talked about is how too much stress can also cause a slowing of the thyroid, called hypothyroidism.

Any kind of stress prompts the brain to release CRH (corticotropin-releasing hormone). But both cortisol and CRH can inhibit TSH and the conversion of T4 to T3, our most active thyroid hormone.

Because every cell in the body uses T3 for healthy function, the decrease in T3 can lead to symptoms like:

- Fatigue
- Poor concentration
- Sluggishness
- Depression
- Lack of libido
- Insomnia
- Weight gain
- Hair fall
- Infertility
- Intolerance to cold

This inhibition of your thyroid and hormone receptors often takes place quietly behind the scenes for months or years without causing overt symptoms. And this is why so many women are caught off-guard when they are diagnosed with a thyroid disorder. They think everything has been going fine and all of a sudden, they feel horrible. The fact is, if you've been experiencing chronic stress over time, the resulting adrenal imbalance, whether overactive or eventually underactive, has also inhibited your thyroid function. Some women can even remain in what we call 'subclinical hypothyroidism', where their thyroid hormone levels are within the standard normal ranges, even while they're experiencing symptoms of low thyroid function.

Our adrenal glands are meant to provide us with the support we need during the perimenopause years, so we have abundant energy and are able to function efficiently through the day. Instead, we see women pushing themselves with stimulants like caffeine, alcohol and sugary foods, which deplete the adrenals, causing them to get exhausted. When this happens, the stress hormones, norepinephrine (adrenaline) and cortisol are over-produced, leading to fatigue. Shonali has gone through adrenal exhaustion personally and she recommends that you help yourself by simply tweaking your food habits and lifestyle.

Here are signs that you could be suffering from adrenal exhaustion:

- You have fat around your belly.
- You find that you do not wake up fresh from sleep in the mornings, maybe suffer from insomnia.
- You feel the need for coffee and tea to get you going in the mornings.
- You find it difficult to fall asleep at night, because you are wired.

- You rely on sugar and sugary foods when you are stressed or feel the need for energy.
- Your libido levels plummet.
- You are foggy in your thinking.
- You have poor memory.
- You suffer frequent headaches.
- You suffer mood swings.

Snapshot on Lifestyle and Diet

- Keep stress levels under control by using techniques like meditation, yoga, pranayama—any practice that might work for you.
- Support your adrenal function by resting and relaxing a lot.
- Exercise to increase endorphins.
- Make sure a whole grain (brown rice/millet) is a part of your diet.
- Avoid soy as it may lower your body's ability to take in benefits of medication.
- Avoid sugar, alcohol and refined flour, anything that would cause the sugar response of the body to go out of balance.
- Avoid intermittent fasting and fasting in general, as this is likely to deplete the adrenals.
- Include seaweed like spirulina for hypothyroidism since it supplies you with iodine. This is to be avoided in hyperthyroidism.
- If you are using supplements, consult your health practitioner as they may interfere with your thyroid medication.
- Selenium from whole grains and nuts can help with a malfunctioning thyroid.

- Add shilajit to your diet, as it has minerals that help increase thyroid function.
- Add vitamin-C-rich foods as it supports your blood vessels.
- Add magnesium as it helps with the utilization of energy by the body.
- Make sure your vitamin-D levels are within range and if not supplement it.
- It is a myth that you should avoid cruciferous vegetables like cauliflower, broccoli and cabbage as they have goitrogens. These get inactivated as soon as they are cooked.
- Slow down your eating process and give the thyroid a chance to record the message that you are eating.
- Keep your cell phone away when eating.
- The thyroid gland is connected to the voice, your centre of communication, so if you suffer from hyperthyroid learn to quieten down; but with hypothyroid, speak up.
- Improve sleep hygiene; make sure you sleep deep and well.

What Are the Immunizations Recommended during the Perimenopause?

Immunization has a particularly important protective role in the perimenopause. There are certain vaccines that are now considered essential and required vaccines should be discussed with your doctor. The recommended vaccines for perimenopausal women include the following:

- **Influenza** Annual influenza shots are recommended to all women aged fifty years and older.

- **Tetanus diphtheria** Tetanus diphtheria (Td) booster is recommended every ten years. Age fifty is a good time to get a booster vaccination if you cannot remember when your last one was. Because of a resurgence of pertussis (whooping cough), a single dose of Tdap vaccine is recommended for unvaccinated adults under the age of sixty-four years.
- **Pneumonia** Everyone over the age of sixty-five years should receive this immunization once. Patients with diseases such as diabetes, malignancies or steroid therapy, should receive it more often.
- **Varicella (chickenpox)** If you have never had chickenpox, a two-dose series is advisable.
- **Shingles** Indicated for women who have already had chickenpox but not shingles and are aged over fifty years.
- **Meningitis, hepatitis A, hepatitis B** For peri- and post-menopausal women travelling to exotic locations, certain vaccinations such as meningococcal and hepatitis (A and B) should be considered.

4

What to Expect: Clinical Situations and Solutions

'Health is not valued till sickness comes.'

—Thomas Fuller

This section is like an SOP (Standard Operating Procedure) manual for women. We start with menstrual symptoms and then touch upon some of the common associated problems such as benign breast disease, fibroids and endometriosis that you could face during the perimenopause. Read this as a precursor to Section 2, in which we will approach in detail the various perimenopausal problems listed in the Menopause Rating Scale (MRS), with their presentations and solutions.

The Modified Menopause Rating Scale

The MRS was designed and standardized as a self-administered scale to assess the symptoms/complaints of ageing women, to evaluate the severity of symptoms over time and to measure response to treatment. Based on this scale we have created a modified self-test so as to know the types, extent and severity of your symptoms so that you can make the best use of this book. We have also matched the symptoms with chapters you can directly reference.

It is a closed-ended scheme of answering based on rating each symptom you experience. You assign a score from zero to four—with zero being no symptoms at four being severely experienced symptoms. The total score is a sum of the scores (number) you assign to each symptom you are experiencing.

Which of the following symptoms apply to you at this time?

Symptoms Self-assigned score Chapter to reference	None 0	Mild 1	Moderate 2	Severe 3	Very Severe 4
Vasomotor issues Hot flushes and night sweats Profuse sweating **Chapter 5**					
Skin and hair issues Dryness and wrinkling Thinning and hair loss **Chapter 6**					
Vaginal issues Dryness or burning Pain during and after sex **Chapter 7**					

Urinary issues Increased frequency Loss of bladder control Repeated infections **Chapter 7**				
Sexual issues Reduced sex drive Difficulty in reaching orgasm **Chapter 8**				
Joint and muscle issues Joint pains and backache Muscle stiffness and fatigue **Chapter 9**				
Heart issues Palpitations and racing heart Chest discomfort **Chapter 10**				
Sleep issues Difficulty falling asleep Disturbed sleep **Chapter 11**				
Anxiety and anger issues Irrational worry and panic Irritability and hypersensitivity **Chapter 11**				

Depression issues Feeling sad and weepy Mood swings **Chapter 11**					
Cognitive issues Decreased mental ability Lack of concentration Forgetfulness and memory loss **Chapter 11**					

Interpretation of scoring of symptoms to assess severity of menopause

Menopausal State	None or Mild	Mild	Moderate	Severe
Scores	0–4	5–8	9–16	17+

Abnormal Bleeding Patterns in the Perimenopause

You may have disturbed menstrual cycles in the run up to menopause, swinging between periods being too light or too heavy, coming too late and sometimes early. There are medical terms for these conditions, and it is important to know these to understand the changes as they unfold.

- **Amenorrhea** is when there are no periods. This happens because estrogen levels fall below the level needed to grow the uterine lining, the endometrium.
- **Hypomenorrhea** is where the periods are scanty. This happens because the endometrium does not get adequate

stimulus due to low levels of estrogen or where there is endometrial damage due to infection or injury.

- **Menorrhagia** is where the periods are too heavy and often with clots. This happens because the endometrium responds to fluctuating estrogen levels, which are sometimes high. The endometrium becomes too thick (hyperplasia) and may develop endometrial polyps.
- **Metrorrhagia** is where there is bleeding or spotting between periods. This could be because of fluctuating estrogen levels or endometrial polyps which cause intermittent breakdown or shedding of the endometrial lining.
- **Polymenorrhagia** is where the periods are too frequent. The follicular phase shortens although the luteal phase remains constant, leading to shorter more frequent cycles.
- **Oligomenorrhea** is where the periods are less frequent. This is because of absent ovulation (anovulation) which leads to delayed irregular cycles.
- **Dysmenorrhea** is where the periods are painful. This may be primary without an obvious cause or secondary because of associated conditions such as endometriosis and adenomyosis.

Over 90 per cent of women have regular periods until the age of forty years. Between the ages of forty to fifty only 10 per cent will have normal cycles, with about 25 per cent bleeding heavily during this phase. So it is quite normal to face a situation of irregularity in your periods in the run up to menopause.

The reasons for menstrual disturbances are as follows:

- When estrogen levels are lower, the uterine lining gets thinner and the flow is lighter and scanty.
- When there is more estrogen which is not balanced by progestogen because of anovulation, the uterine lining overgrows and bleeding is heavier.
- When the early part of the follicular phase (the first half of the cycle) becomes shorter, the periods are more frequent. The number of days from the day your period begins to the day you ovulate can vary to anywhere between three to fourteen days of your cycle, while the number of days from ovulation to the next period remains constant at about fourteen days.

It is normal, in a way, to face menstrual irregularities in the pre-menopause phase. Women going through menopause are often deficient in progesterone. As the body stops ovulating and the uterine lining does not shed efficiently, irregularity in your periods signals this deficiency. The shedding of the endometrium lining is stimulated by the fall of progesterone levels about fifteen days post ovulation. As a result of not ovulating every month, you will face irregular periods.

To manage abnormal bleeding patterns doctors will generally offer the following treatments:

- For irregular periods, cyclic progestogens given ten to fifteen days a month or oral contraceptive pills (COCs) regularize periods. There is also the recent concept of adjusting or extending COC use to even up to eighty-four days to allow women control over their periods and their lives.
- For heavy periods, tranexamic acid given during the period reduces flow significantly. The levonorgestrel

Figure 4: The influence of estrogen levels on menstrual regularity or irregularity

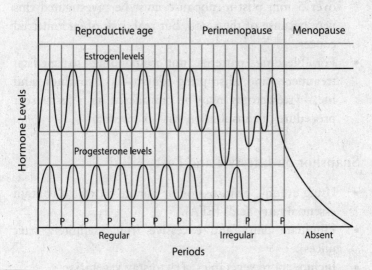

intrauterine system (Mirena), a progestogen releasing intrauterine device can be used both for contraception and to reduce bleeding by 90 per cent over time. Endometrial ablation and transcervical resection of the endometrium (TCRE), where the roots of the endometrium are excised, is a minimally invasive, day-care alternative to hysterectomy.

- For painful periods, anti-prostaglandins like mefenamic acid or anti-inflammatory medication like ibuprofen reduce pain significantly. Here too there is a role for endometrial ablation and TCRE, particularly in the presence of adenomyosis, where the uterine lining grows into the muscle of the uterine wall.
- For endometrial hyperplasia, hysteroscopy is used to assess the uterine cavity and a dilatation and curettage

(D&C) is then performed to remove the uterine lining, which is then sent for pathology testing. Any thickness over 5 mm post-menopause must be investigated this way because of the small, but real, risk of endometrial cancer.

- For bleeding patterns not responding to medical treatment and disrupting day-to-day routines and life, hysterectomy may be considered as a last-resort procedure in consultation with the woman.

Snapshot on Lifestyle and Diet

- Using evening primrose oil or borage oil which contain essential fatty acids (EFA).
- Eliminate dairy and excessive fruit (definitely fruit juices).
- Include more vegetables. Try to stay vegetarian.
- Avoid caffeine, sugar, refined flour (maida), processed and packaged foods.
- Add a good multivitamin.
- Taking magnesium helps keep progesterone in check.
- Add chia or flax seeds.
- Liquorice root tea helps.
  - Ingredients are 2 tsp of liquorice root, 1 cup of water and honey to taste.
  - Boil the water, add the liquorice root, steep for 5 to 6 minutes.
  - Strain and drink warm.

Why Is There Weight Gain in the Perimenopause?

My own story is a classic example of weight gain in the perimenopause. I have always had a carrom-board tummy; I have a pretty intense workout routine and also swim regularly, and I have an optimum diet. Yet, during these years, two things have happened: I have gained 3 to 4 kilos, and my tummy is no longer a carrom board.

Tennessee Williams said, 'There comes a time when you look into the mirror and you realize that what you see is all that you will ever be. And then you accept it. Or kill yourself. Or you stop looking in mirrors.'

That's what I did with my tummy bulge. I stopped looking in the mirror and accepted my situation as it is. It is normal to gain some weight during this time, as it is the body's coping mechanism to what is coming—your menopause. The hips, thighs, buttocks and abdomen, where all the fatty tissue of women really is, will tend to harbour some more fat; this fat actually is a protection for us. The fat cells begin to produce more estrogen as the ovarian production of estrogen declines. It is best then to stop worrying and start living.

In the meantime, I have doubled my efforts to take care of my diet and exercise. The body has the tendency to crave when there are hormonal imbalances. This is especially true for caffeine, sugar and white carbs when the energy hits a low. These foods are considered stimulants and will push your adrenal function into an overdrive situation. It's better to be mindful of this happening than to give in to these foods. Of course, you must not put on too much weight, so be mindful of this as well. Why you must keep a sharp lookout for excess weight gain (anything above 3 to 4 kilos) is because this will then set the body up for insulin resistance, a place you do not want to get to. Also, we do not need stress at this time, as that will push cortisol levels up as well.

Shonali Sabherwal

Weight gain at midlife is often attributed to hormonal changes at menopause. However, studies have shown this not to be the case. The steady weight gain of about 0.5 kg per year seen in women at midlife is associated with age and environmental factors, not menopause. Disruption of the day-night circadian rhythm by work and sleep deprivation also contributes to weight gain. The relationship between depression and midlife weight gain goes both ways.

Still, the change in the hormonal environment at this time is associated with significant increases in waist circumference and central abdominal fat. The redistribution of fat to the abdomen results in a transition from a gynoid to an android pattern of fat distribution. Waist circumference represents both subcutaneous and visceral adipose tissue deposit size and correlates closely with cardiovascular disease risk and abnormal lipids.

Weight management and prevention of weight gain are essential components in the care of post-menopausal women. Optimizing body weight should be considered early in the perimenopause to safeguard the quality of life. The primary approach to weight management should be encouragement of a healthy diet and physical activity. Management of factors associated with weight gain such as depression is important. If depression requires medical treatment, medications associated with weight gain such as clozapine, imipramine and amitriptyline should be avoided if possible.

Contrary to widespread belief, menopause hormone therapy (MHT) is not associated with weight gain and may instead ameliorate accumulation of abdominal fat, improve insulin sensitivity and help with lower rate of development of type-2 diabetes. Oral estrogen may be associated with a small but significant increase in fat mass and a decrease in lean mass, whereas these are unaffected by transdermal estradiol.

Snapshot on Lifestyle and Diet

- Exercise, including both cardio and strength, Pilates, weight training or functional.
- Be regular with mealtimes.
- Regulate sleep habits.
- Avoid sugar, yeasted foods, alcohol, stimulants like coffee, sodas, colas and teas.
- Eliminate simple carbohydrates and all junk foods.
- Increase the consumption of complex carbohydrates (within limits—say, 50 grams of cooked carbs at breakfast, 100 grams at lunch and 50 to 80 grams at

dinner) like brown rice and millets as this will not only aid the digestive system, but also help flush out extra unwanted fats in the system.

- Add all legumes and lentils.
- Add 1 to 2 tablespoons chia or flax seeds a day to your diet for Omega 3.
- Include some probiotics via foods like kanji, pressed salads, quick pickles, kefir and miso paste.
- Make your diet the cornerstone of sorting the weight gain.

What Is the Significance of Painful Breasts?

Estimates point at 70 per cent of women experiencing painful breasts or mastalgia at one time or another in their journey to menopause. Fibrocystic breast disease is where cysts or tender lumps form in the breast because of hormonal changes causing fluid build-up, making breasts feel swollen and tender. Unopposed estrogen, which may happen to women at the time around perimenopause, would lead to retaining both salt and water, increasing fibrocystic breasts.

Breast pain around menopause may also feel different. Instead of a dull ache, women may experience burning or throbbing pain. Cysts, if present, may be painful. Since they feel like lumps, they may induce concern, given that breast cancer is now so prevalent. Be reassured that sore and painful breasts, while uncomfortable, are generally not likely to be associated with cancer.

If there are any of the following symptoms in addition to sore breasts, you should see a doctor:

- Noticeable changes in the size and shape of breasts, particularly if they occur only on one side.

- Changes and thickening in skin texture.
- Unexplained discharge from the nipple.
- Swelling or lump in the armpit or around the collarbone.
- Lump or abnormally firm area on the breast.

To manage painful breasts:

- Wear supportive bras that fit comfortably, avoiding the compression caused by underwired bras.
- Exercise regularly.
- Use an anti-inflammatory like ibuprofen to treat sore breasts.
- When in pain, avoid wearing a bra and apply a warm compress.
- Take a hot shower.
- Take a multivitamin, vitamin E 400 IU, magnesium 400 mg and B6 100 mg.
- Perform a self-examination and also get a breast examination done periodically.

Snapshot on Lifestyle and Diet

- Wear a comfortable, supportive bra with a good fit.
- Cut back on alcohol.
- Give up caffeine, which includes colas and sodas.
- Quit smoking.
- Reduce salt consumption to reduce fluid retention.
- Cut back bad quality fat, which means there should be no trans fats, found in hydrogenated vegetable oil used in packaged foods. Cut back on fat in general will also help.
- Give up dairy products, as unassimilated casein will add to the risk of forming cysts in the breasts.

- Increase the consumption of complex carbohydrates like brown rice and millets as this will not only aid the digestive system but also help flush out extra unwanted fats in the system.
- Add 1–2 tablespoons chia or flax seeds a day to your diet for Omega 3.
- Use a liver-support formula.
- Use amalaki (amla or gooseberry powder).
- Black currant seed or borage oil which has gamma-linoleic acid and Omega 6 fatty acid.

How Do You Cope with Acid Reflux and Heartburn?

Stomach acid, both the excess or lack of it, can create a host of issues affecting gut diversity. Stomach acid makes food more digestible and kills microbes. It tends to decrease when your health is compromised or you are under stress. When there is not enough acid, food remains undigested, making it unable to pass on to the small intestine, making you prone to acid reflux and heartburn. Acid reflux is when the stomach acid is pushed back up the oesophagus and you experience a burning sensation in your chest and a sour taste in your mouth.

Many perimenopausal and menopausal women manifest symptoms of acid reflux with uncomfortable burning, upper abdominal pain and bloating or, if they had mild symptoms before, these get significantly worse. It is estimated that menopausal women are three times more likely to suffer from gastroesophageal reflux disease (GERD). As a result of fluctuating hormone levels, estrogen and progesterone imbalances can cause the rhythmic muscular activity within the gut to be disrupted, resulting in digestive problems.

Besides this, cortisol can cause stress-induced tummy ache and changes in FSH can promote feelings of nausea. Falling estrogen levels can affect the production of acid in the stomach and when this happens you can start to experience indigestion, wind and feeling of fullness, with a lot of the discomfort and pain.

In many cases there is an imbalance in the consumption of protein and carbohydrates, with refined carbohydrates being predominant. In such a scenario there is an overproduction of inflammatory substances which will suppress immune function, increase stomach issues and increase inflammation in your digestive system. High blood sugar impacts secretion of gastric juices and any refined carbohydrates will set the stage for indigestion.

The management of gastritis and GERD is a combination of lifestyle modification, diet and medical treatment. Lifestyle modification should be initiated and continued throughout the course of therapy. While the occasional use of antacids by self-medication is justified, persistent symptoms need longer-term treatment and a doctor should be consulted:

- Antacids are effective in relieving GERD symptoms, with less acid regurgitation and fewer days and nights with heartburn. Many women try to address gastric issues by resorting to self-medication with over-the-counter antacids, with a third using antacids twice a week. Antacids with aluminium hydroxide neutralize stomach acid, but cause constipation and with prolonged use reduce phosphate levels resulting in fatigue and loss of appetite. Those with magnesium hydroxide can cause diarrhoea. Those with calcium carbonate cause acid rebound, a condition in which the excess calcium actually stimulates increased acid secretion. Chronic calcium carbonate intake is associated with a pattern of blood chemistry known as milk alkali syndrome, producing elevations of calcium, phosphate and bicarbonate with development of kidney stones over time.

- Histamine2-receptor antagonists (H2RA) such as cimetidine, ranitidine and famotidine on prescription are effective in relieving heartburn in patients with GERD in up to 70 per cent of women. Some women with GERD may be able to predict when they will have reflux symptoms and may benefit from premedication.

- Proton pump inhibitors (PPI) such as omeprazole, pantoprazole and rabeprazole are the step-up therapy if there is poor response to H2RA therapy. Esomeprazole (Nexium) is an isomer of omeprazole and is associated with higher rates of healing and symptom resolution. Side effects include headache and diarrhoea and a reduction in vitamin B12 absorption.

- You may be checked for *Helicobacter pylori*. Antibiotic medications are prescribed if *H. pylori* is diagnosed in your digestive tract. Be sure to take the full antibiotic prescription, usually for seven to fourteen days, along with medication to block acid production.

Snapshot on Lifestyle and Diet

- Hydrate with 2–2½ litres of fluids in a day.
- Eat three main meals and two small snacks in the day.
- Avoid lying down within three to four hours after a meal. Have your last meal of the day three hours before bedtime.
- Elevate the head of the bed by 10–20 cm.

- Eat low gastrointestinal glycaemic index foods.
- Add fermented foods to aid good gut bacteria.
- Always include a protein as a snack.
- Eliminate white refined flour from your diet.
- Take vitamin C and E supplement.
- Take a calcium and magnesium or supplement your diet with spirulina and kombu.
- Be judicious with antacid use since they reduce stomach acid, which you need to absorb vitamin B12. You are at risk of vitamin B12 deficiency if you overuse antacids.
- Take a good digestive enzyme.
- Take 60 ml of aloe vera juice in your daily protein shakes.
- Make a tea with fennel, anise and chamomile to ease any gas or bloating.

What Is the Issue with PCOS at the Perimenopause?

Women with PCOS tend to reach menopause about two years later than the average age. Since PCOS does not go away with menopause, symptoms may continue. In fact, many symptoms of PCOS such as irregular or missed periods, weight gain and insulin resistance, acne and skin problems are similar to those of perimenopause, which may make it difficult for women to be newly diagnosed. PCOS and menopause are both related to anovulation and affect the levels of progesterone which is why menopause does not treat or cure PCOS.

Management of PCOS at the perimenopause depends on what your complaints are:

- To regulate your menstrual cycle, your doctor may recommend birth-control pills (COCs).

- To regulate your menstrual cycle your doctor may also recommend progestin therapy.
- To help you with ovulation and to conceive, your doctor may also recommend oral anti-estrogen medication in the first part of your menstrual cycle.
- A popular medication is metformin which is for type 2 diabetic patients to improve insulin resistance.
- If you have excessive hair growth, antiandrogens are the first-line treatment. The medical treatment is then complemented by hair removal using laser treatments or electrolysis.

Snapshot on Lifestyle and Diet

- Make healthier food choices, as outlined in the diet section of the book and definitely control the insulin response.
- Limiting carbs at this time would help considerably.
- Get your weight down if you are overweight.
- Exercise to lose weight.
- Up your magnesium.
- Inositol is a sugar alcohol once considered Vitamin B8 that may help with insulin resistance.
- Cinnamon has been proved to have a positive effect on insulin. You can make water infused with cinnamon and sip it throughout the day.
- Add zinc to boost the immune system and combat excessive hair growth.
- Turmeric, which has been shown to improve immunity, is an anti-inflammatory and helps with insulin resistance.
- Evening primrose oil will help with cholesterol, period pain and irregular menstruation, decreasing oxidative stress.

- Women with PCOS usually have low levels of vitamin D so supplementation will help and along with calcium, it may help with irregular periods.
- Omega 3 fatty acids in cod liver oil or chia and flax seeds will help regulate periods.
- Ashwagandha helps balance cortisol levels.
- Maca root is a traditional herb used to balance hormones and lower cortisol.
- Tulsi (holy basil) will help reduce blood sugar and address metabolic stress, reducing blood-sugar levels.
- Liquorice root contains a compound called glycyrrhizin which is an anti-inflammatory, helping to balance hormones.
- Chaga mushroom tea boosts immunity, supports immune system and fights inflammation, which most people suffering with PCOS have. It also enhances liver health to clear out toxins and balance blood-sugar levels.

Why Are Fibroids Still an Issue during the Perimenopause?

I remember my first encounter with fibroids (non-cancerous lumps that grow in the uterus) when twenty years ago my friend, Lynn, was diagnosed with one (the size of a lemon) and I had to help her decide on an alternative course of action. Luckily it was not big enough, so homeopathy sorted her out. My second encounter was with my friend, Dilnavaz, who had a larger fibroid (described as the size of a musk melon) and she just stayed with it. I remember her telling me that when her first baby was born, it was huge and since she had a C-section, the priority was the baby, so the doctors just pushed her fibroid back in. She still has it and has had a second baby.

Shonali Sabherwal

P worked with my wife and is a dear friend to us. She is unmarried, a wonderful daughter and friend and an achiever with next level sincerity and dedication. She first came to me for a routine check when she was forty years old. She had multiple uterine fibroids, not uncommon for her profile, with no symptoms, so we decided to leave the fibroids alone and just monitor them annually. At the age of forty-six, P came to me in distress, having a meltdown. She had gone for a corporate health check where she was told her fibroids had increased in size and that she should undergo a removal of her uterus at the earliest. The justification was that she was forty-six years old and unmarried so she did not have any need for her uterus, a decision that should have been hers not the doctor's. I did find that her uterus was much larger, measuring 18 x 12 x 10 cm on ultrasound, almost the size of a pregnancy at five months. She had many fibroids, the largest being 9 cm, followed by some measuring 8 cm, 5 cm and 3 cm, all in or outside the uterine wall. She had absolutely no symptoms and her FSH level was seven, so menopause was sometime away. Now you never treat a report, you treat the person and we decided together to continue to be conservative in our approach. We now had ulipristal to treat fibroids medically and we decided to use this treatment with close monitoring of her liver function, which in rare instances, is known to be negatively impacted by ulipristal. She stayed on ulipristal for three years, with her uterus shrinking in size by a third, at which time the medication was stopped. P reached menopause a year ago and her uterus is now down to 11 x 9 x 6 cm. She always remembers the day she met me in panic and remains thankful that she avoided surgery.

A woman must be part of all decision-making and where medically feasible must be allowed her own choices. Her doctor should see things from her perspective and help her with treatments that she is comfortable with, even if it means pushing clinical boundaries. P's regular follow ups continue, and we look forward to her visits accompanied by her frail, charming and adorable mother.

Nozer Sheriar

Fibroids or myomas are the most common types of benign tumours in women. Uterine fibroids increase with age, reaching an incidence of over 50 per cent in women aged fifty years. While they develop most often in women of childbearing age, they continue to affect women during and after menopause or even develop for the first time during this stage of life. After menopause, since the body produces less estrogen and progesterone the risk of new fibroids decreases and the drop in hormone levels may also help pre-existing fibroids decrease in size.

Most fibroids cause few or no symptoms. Depending on size, number and location, others may result in heavy and painful periods (submucous fibroids in the uterine cavity), interfere with conception and pregnancy and large or multiple fibroids may put pressure on internal organs such as the bladder causing frequent urination (intramural fibroids within the wall or subserous fibroids on the surface of the uterus).

Treating fibroids during the perimenopause is nuanced and must be individualized:

- For asymptomatic fibroids, even large ones, no active treatment is required and watchful expectancy where ultrasound checks are done periodically (say, six-monthly), is offered and practised.
- For fibroids causing symptoms, these may be conserved and the symptoms managed with COCs, tranexamic acid and mefenamic acid as discussed earlier. If the uterine cavity is normal, the progestogen-releasing-intrauterine device (Mirena) can also be used.
- For large fibroids, medical treatment is now a reality with the use of ulipristal acetate and mifepristone, which can reduce the size by a third and alleviate symptoms. There are concerns about the effect of ulipristal on the liver so its use must be monitored closely.
- For submucous fibroids, particularly those causing menstrual problems or infertility, hysteroscopic myomectomy, the excision of fibroids within the cavity using an operative telescope through the vagina and the cervix, is now the favoured treatment and cure.

- For large or multiple intramural or subserous fibroids, causing pressure symptoms or infertility, surgical removal by myomectomy either by open surgery or minimally invasive laparoscopic surgery.
- For fibroids that are large, symptomatic or recur after previous surgery, for women in the perimenopause, where they do not plan further children and where they are willing to undergo definitive surgery, a hysterectomy (the surgical removal of the uterus) may be performed after adequate counselling. This may be by vaginal hysterectomy, abdominal hysterectomy or laparoscopic hysterectomy.
- Wherever possible the ovaries must be retained since ovarian function continues and protects women until and even after menopause sets in.

Snapshot on Lifestyle and Diet

- Apart from diet, please know that it is your inner ecosystem that has caused a fibroid as well, that is primarily all the foods you have ingested that have not been assimilated that add to the issue.
- Focus on all the gut-building foods in the diet section, improve liver function, reduce gut and overall inflammation in the body and increase lymphatic drainage.
- Minimize endocrine disruptors (read the section again on exposure to xenoestrogens).
- Definitely do not neglect your greens (which maybe in the form of a powder or simply juicing them).
- Improve gut motility.
- Exercise including both cardio and strength (Pilates, yoga, weight training or functional).

- Be regular with mealtimes.
- Regulate sleep habits.
- Homeopathy for fibroids that are not very large, has shown results.
- Craniosacral therapy or even acupuncture will help shrink the size.
- Practise intermittent fasting.

Why Has Endometriosis Become an Important Contemporary Issue?

Endometriosis is a chronic inflammatory condition dependent on estrogen, where the endometrial cells from the uterine lining implant and grow outside the normal cavity of the uterus. This could be on the outside surface of the uterus, on or within the ovaries, where they may result in chocolate cysts, or on the fallopian tubes and other organs, such as the bladder and rectum. Endometriosis reacts to every menstrual cycle and the hormones, with local bleeding and the tissue swelling up, causing pain and bleeding in the areas that they are lodged into. It is estimated to occur in between 5 and 10 per cent of women of reproductive age. While post-menopausal endometriosis is rare, because of the reduction or absence of estrogen production, it is a problem women face during the perimenopause. Reactivation of endometriosis can occur in some post-menopausal women, either as a side effect of therapy with administered hormones or because of the presence of estrogen from other sources. The prevalence of post-menopausal endometriosis is 2 to 5 per cent.

Endometriosis can be extremely painful, and the pain will start manifesting ten to twelve days before your period, and then get worse as the menstrual cycle continues. With adenomyosis, where the endometriosis is in the uterine muscle, period cycles would be heavy and painful. Endometriosis will cause pain during intercourse as well.

Although the exact cause of endometriosis is not certain, possible explanations include:

- Retrograde menstruation where endometrial cells carried in menstrual blood flows back through the fallopian tubes and out into the pelvic cavity; these cells stick to the surfaces of pelvic organs, where they grow and continue to thicken and bleed over the course of each menstrual cycle.
- Transformation of peritoneal and embryonic cells in which hormones or immune factors promote transformation of peritoneal cells into endometrial-like cells.
- Endometrial cell transported by blood vessels or lymphatic system to other parts of the body.
- Immune system disorder that makes the body unable to recognize and destroy endometrial-like tissue that grow outside the uterus.

While the cause of endometriosis is unclear, as already mentioned, exposure to environmental toxins has a big role to play and minimizing exposure to them could be a good start towards prevention.

Xenoestrogens, environmental toxins that behave like estrogen (endocrine disruptors), are a major contemporary problem leading to hormonal imbalances. Endocrine disruptors mimic hormones and in doing so will bind to hormone receptors:

- Polychlorinated biphenyls (PCBs) (used as coolants, transformers, capacitors and other, usually electrical, equipment because they are good insulators that don't burn easily) are linked to breast cancer.
- Parabens (used as a preservative in the pharmaceutical and cosmetic industry) are linked to menstrual irregularity.
- Poly and perfluoroalkyl substances (PFAs) (usually found in the coating of our pans for their thermal and chemical resistant properties) lead to menstrual irregularity.
- Bisphenol A (BPA) (found in plastic) has links to PCOS.
- Phthalate (substances added to plastic) have links to PCOS and fibroids.

It should be your goal to identify and reduce the endocrine disruptors in your life and do the following:

- Reduce exposure by removing all these products from your household.
- Be a discerning consumer by constantly looking for eco-friendly alternatives.
- Use detoxification via panchakarma, massages or saunas to get rid of toxins built up within you.
- Make sure your liver is functioning well and aid it in the detoxification process by eating fibre and using leafy-green vegetable juice.

While endometriosis may cause few or no symptoms, depending on stage, location and duration, it may manifest symptoms, from mild to severe. At its worst it can incapacitate women's lives.

Diagnosis of endometriosis has always been a challenge:

- The classic symptoms are pelvic pain, painful menses and painful sex before and during the period.
- During a pelvic exam there will be pain, scarring behind the uterus and ovarian cysts.
- CA 125 is a marker that is elevated in endometriosis.
- Ultrasound can identify chocolate cysts.
- Magnetic resonance imaging (MRI) can identify ovarian cysts, endometrial implants and rectal endometriosis.
- Laparoscopy is the gold standard since the diagnosis is visual.

Treatment of endometriosis could be conservative, medical or surgical:

- Pain medication such as the non-steroidal anti-inflammatory drugs (NSAIDs) ibuprofen or naproxen to help ease painful menstrual cramps.
- Hormone therapy to slow endometrial tissue growth and prevent new implants of endometrial tissue. These include oral contraceptive pills, progestogens such as dinogest and injections of depot medroxyprogesterone acetate (DMPA) and injections of gonadotrophin releasing hormone (GnRH) to induce temporary menopause.
- Conservative surgery to remove the endometriosis implants while preserving your uterus and ovaries, usually by laparoscopy.
- Hysterectomy with removal of the ovaries as a last resort for severe endometriosis and/or adenomyosis.

Snapshot on Lifestyle and Diet

- Minimize exposure to xenoestrogens, toxic environmental pollutants.
- Exercise including both cardio and strength (Pilates, yoga, weight training or functional).
- Be regular with mealtimes.
- Regulate sleep habits.
- Keep stress under control.
  - Excessive cortisol under stress will aggravate inflammation which will harm the skin.
  - Also causing sugar cravings, which is the worst situation to be in for skin health.
- Many skincare products contain endocrine-disrupting chemicals (EDCs); these interfere with proper hormonal functioning; instead of helping, these get absorbed into the skin, causing problems. So, know the products you are using. Some things to watch out for are parabens, oxybenzone (sunscreens) and products that have perfume.
- Practise meditation (to combat estrogen dominance) and pranayama (nothing like being calm).

Part Two

Deconstructing Clinical Situations and Understanding Treatment Options

'Health is a state of complete harmony of the body, mind and spirit.'

—B.K.S. Iyengar

5

Hot Flushes, Night Sweats and Vasomotor Disturbance

'Sunrise paints the sky with pinks and the sunset with peaches. Cool to warm. So is the progression to old age.'
—Vera Nazarian

At least three out of five of my friends complained of hot flushes in the pre-menopause phase and some still go through them post-menopause. My friend, Lynn, said that in the thick of a New York winter, she kicks off her duvet and sleeps without anything for a cover, as she is drenched in sweat. She has ultimately taken to a gel mattress. Because they can go on for years, hot flushes can cause much distress in a woman's life. They result in intense heat in your extremities, profuse sweating and even heart palpitations. They usually come in surges and are not long in duration, usually lasting between five to ten minutes. As we approach our menopause, these flushes tend to get more intense.

Shonali Sabherwal

K first met me when she was forty-two years old. She had this wonderful positive temperament, exercised regularly and was amazingly fit. Suddenly her otherwise settled life was majorly disrupted by distressing, uncontrolled bouts of flushes and sweating. She was still menstruating with irregular periods, but her FSH levels were thirty-four, suggesting that her symptoms were clearly perimenopausal. After workup and counselling, she started on menopause hormone therapy (MHT) with estrogen patches and progesterone and her symptoms magically vanished in a few weeks. Now, a woman with hot flushes who is suddenly relieved of them considers her doctor a magician, but it is really the estrogens that are the magician's prop. K continued the MHT for four years, then shifting to tibolone for twelve more years. Hormone therapy made the disappearance of symptoms seem almost magical and K, whom we call Mrs Sunshine in our practice, continues to be a patient and a dear friend twenty-two years on.

Nozer Sheriar

The Dynamic Reactive Vasomotor System

The vasomotor system is a network of small blood vessels under the skin. As per the situation, these can dilate, relax and fill with blood or constrict, narrow and restrict blood flow. When the vessels are dilated, the skin is flushed, red and warm; and when the vessels are constricted, the skin is pale and cold.

Symptoms such as flushing, sweating, palpitations and even chills are amongst the earliest and most dramatic symptoms that women experience in perimenopause. They are generally the most common reason for women to seek care and request MHT. Since they result from disruptions in the response of the small blood vessels below the skin, they are called vasomotor symptoms (VMS). While VMS are medically harmless, they are uncomfortable and distressing with a major impact on day-to-day activities. These symptoms are very common in menopausal transition, affecting approximately four out of ten women in the perimenopause and six to eight out of ten women immediately before and then in the post menopause.

VMS present as a hot flash, that is, a feeling of intense heat on the face, arms and upper body, which is then followed by a hot flush, which is a flushing of the skin in the affected areas and profuse sweating. Flashes and flushes are often accompanied by palpitations, giddiness, anxiety and a feeling of weakness.

What Causes Hot Flushes?

While the exact reason for VMS is incompletely understood, they are related to a disturbed temperature-control mechanism in perimenopausal women's bodies.

Figure 5: Skin changes during and after hot flushes

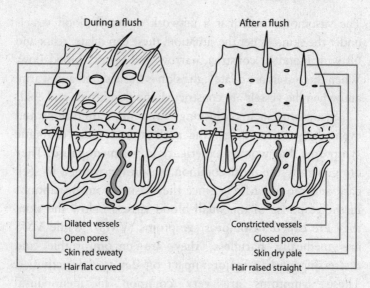

During a flush

After a flush

- Dilated vessels
- Open pores
- Skin red sweaty
- Hair flat curved

- Constricted vessels
- Closed pores
- Skin dry pale
- Hair raised straight

The part of the brain called the hypothalamus is responsible for controlling our body's core temperature. It maintains a thermoneutral zone which allows the body to withstand a reasonable range of temperatures without triggering responses to lose heat, such as the relaxation of the blood vessels below the skin and sweating. The drop in levels or withdrawal of estrogen that happens in the perimenopause triggers VMS by increasing two substances—norepinephrine and serotonin. This narrows the thermoneutral zone so that very small increases in core temperature trigger dilatation of blood vessels and sweating to lose heat and small decreases in temperature trigger shivers and chills to retain heat. It is these magnified and wild swings in the way vessels behave that causes the disruptive VMS. The onset of a flush has also been found to coincide with an elevation in the luteinizing hormone (LH) secreted by the pituitary gland. Interestingly, it is the drop in estrogen levels that causes these symptoms and not just low estrogen levels, since women with chronic very low estrogen levels because of premature ovarian insufficiency do not experience VMS.

While every woman has a different reaction to VMS, an objective classification has been suggested to assess the severity of hot flashes and night sweats:

1. Not present.
2. Mild—Do not interfere with usual activities.
3. Moderate—Interfere somewhat with usual activities.
4. Severe—So bothersome that usual activities cannot be performed.

VMS not only disturb women and interrupt their day-to-day activities, the night sweats disrupt sleep, causing emotional lability and difficulty concentrating.

VMS are finally self-limiting, reaching maximum intensity during the first two years' post-menopause and then declining over time. Hot flushes generally last for six months to two years, although some women may experience them for ten years or longer.

Snapshot on Lifestyle and Diet

Lifestyle Recommendations

- Establish regularity in meals and be relentless about this. It is okay to slip up two days of the week but try stick to this 85 per cent of the time.

- Recuperate with sleep—this means getting your eight hours of sleep in, or whatever works best.
- Temperature-control your environment by using fans or air-conditioners which most women tend to do at this time. Then get used to one steady temperature.
- Wear lightweight, loose-fitting clothes made with natural fibres such as cotton. This has been a boon for me since I only wear cotton, from my underwear to my clothes.
- Dress in layers, so you can peel them off as required, especially because India is a large country with varying temperatures.
- Again, use cotton sheets and bed covers. Cotton is a fabric that breathes and will always help combat the heat that comes up at this time.
- Add a gel mattress. My friend, Lynn, said this really helped her during her three years pre- and post-menopause, and she is still using it.
- Eliminate stress, since being uncomfortable in the mind upsets the body and its rhythm. Add meditation to your day.
- Take some me-time by adding yoga and movement to get some endorphins going; they will make you feel good.
- Try deep, slow abdominal breathing with six to eight breaths per minute.
  - Practise deep breathing for fifteen minutes in the morning, fifteen minutes in the evening and when a hot flash starts.
- Stay away from bright lights and excessive sunlight.
- Try and quit smoking, because it dehydrates the body and upsets its basal temperature; it also reduces the oxygen supply to the brain.

Diet Recommendations

Please refer to the section in this book on diet for detailed guidance and explanations.

Hot flashes and VMS get aggravated by the foods you eat, as foods have their own energy. When I deal with my clients, I always look at the Ayurvedic classification of body types: vata, pitta and kapha. An aggravated pitta (fire dominant) will make you more prone to VMS and certain foods will aggravate the condition even more. There is always a vata imbalance at this time and foods can play a crucial role in bringing about the balance. By removing pro-inflammatory foods, the dietary recommendations below aim to eliminate or minimize foods that could cause an aggravation of symptoms. Inflammation has become a huge problem, underlying almost all conditions. Macrobiotic philosophy recognizes that eating extreme foods of one nature causes you to attempt to restore the balance by craving extreme foods of the opposite nature.

- Minimize drinking of alcohol and caffeinated drinks. These increase heat in the body.
- Minimize eating spicy foods. These tend to increase sweating, aggravating heat.
- Learn what foods and drinks trigger your hot flashes and limit or completely avoid them as far as possible.
- Sip on cool beverages throughout the day. This could help keep your body temperature down and thereby reduces hot flashes.
- Minimize consuming too much dairy, as dairy does not get totally absorbed by the body. The residue tends to make the blood acidic, causing your basal

temperature to get thrown out of kilter with the acidic load.

- Quit sugar. This includes refined white flour (maida) or off-the-shelf products that have hidden sugars. Sugar plays havoc in your system—it causes an acidic blood condition, robs you of gut bacteria and is what is called a yin food, causing your body to have a mind of its own once you consume it.

- Minimize fruit juices. Fruit is fine, but fruit juices where more than one fruit is used to make a juice are too much fructose for the body to handle and the body treats them as it would sugar.

- Minimize garlic and onion. Both these foods aggravate heat in the body.

- Increase the consumption of complex carbohydrates like brown rice and millets as this will not only aid the digestive system but will keep your sugars steady, bringing in the balance you need.

- Add chia or flax seeds to your diet. The Omega 3 in 1–2 tablespoons a day helps alleviate night sweats.

- Use turmeric as an anti-inflammatory. It will help control all the other negatives that come in when our eating goes haywire during this time; however, use it in moderation. The way we Indians use it in our Indian cooking is adequate.

- Add good fats from avocados, peanuts, olives, nuts and seeds in your diet. These will help combat night sweats.

Medical Management

Be assured that VMSs, however distressing, do not have significant medical implications. These symptoms are generally limited and resolve with time, although this may vary from months to years. While some women learn to live with, and wait out, VMS with no medical treatment and just acceptance and lifestyle modification as outlined earlier, for most others medical treatment is necessary and beneficial.

Hormone Therapy

If the symptoms are bothersome and disruptive, rather than suffering them, you should consult with your doctor about taking estrogens. Estrogen therapy is the gold standard for relief from hot flashes and night sweats and is safe for a short duration until the peak phase of VMS passes. MHT is generally prescribed under medical supervision for a limited time, typically less than five years. While the relief from hot flushes is nothing less than magical, hormone therapy also helps other symptoms such as vaginal dryness and mood disorders. The choice of therapy depends on many factors and has to be individualized. MHT is discussed at length in the chapter on Menopause Hormone Therapy.

- In menstruating perimenopausal women, Combined Oral Contraceptives (COCs) or birth-control pills will control VMS, regularize irregular periods and give the added benefit of reliable birth control. Current practice permits the use of COCs up to the age of fifty years. My preference is to use a low dose COC with drosperinone, which also helps with bloating and PMS-like symptoms.
- A contraceptive patch, if available, is an alternative to COCs and a great option since the hormones bypass the liver.

- If estrogens are to be avoided for medical reasons, then progestogen-only pills may be used at menopause transition for relief of symptoms.
- In post-menopausal women, more natural hormones are used with the combination of hormones used varying, since the uterine lining needs protection from excessive growth.
  o A combined therapy with estrogen and progestogen is used for women with a uterus.
  o Estrogen is used alone for women without a uterus.

Non-Hormonal Medical Treatment

Treatment of VMS without hormones is possible and may be the only option in women where estrogen or progestogen therapy is unsafe or causes side effects. A variety of medications can decrease the frequency and intensity of hot flushes.

- Clonidine is a medication for hypertension used to reduce hot flushes.
- Gabapentin is an anti-convulsant medication specifically useful in patients experiencing nighttime flushes and repeated awakenings. It also has a sedating effect.
- Low-dose anti-depressants are found to improve symptoms in women with mild to moderate hot flushes. Effective antidepressants include venlafaxine, paroxetine and fluoxetine. They can also treat other menopausal symptoms, such as mood swings, anxiety and depression.

Complementary Therapies

While scientific studies have not consistently supported the efficacy of complementary or over-the-counter therapies in reducing severity or frequency of hot flushes or night sweats, many women still find relief with them. As with other supplements, it is important to talk to your doctor before taking these.

- Soya contains large quantities of phytoestrogens, natural chemicals that act like estrogen in the body. It is particularly high in isoflavones, which bind to estrogen receptors and helps reduce hot flashes. Good sources of soya in food are soy milk, tofu, tempeh and edamame. It is believed that Japanese women have a lower incidence of hot flushes and other menopausal symptoms because of the high intake of soya-based products.
- Black cohosh is a popular herb for treating hot flashes and other menopausal symptoms. The root of the plant is used in capsules and less commonly in tea. Although the exact mechanism action is unknown, it is believed to bind to estrogen receptors or stimulate serotonin receptors.
- The use of acupuncture has been shown to have some benefit.
- Hypnosis has been shown to reduce the frequency of VMS and improve sleep quality.

Headaches in the Perimenopause

All my adult life I have had migraines, that is, until I became a macrobiotic nutritionist and cleaned up my lifestyle and diet. But recently a client came to me with a peculiar headache, one that occurred every day for the past six years. The headaches occurred on one side of her head and only for a duration ranging from one to four hours, usually at night and usually at the same time every night. The intensity of the headache—on a scale of 1 to 10, with 10 being the highest—always averaged at a five. For my client, these headaches had started after the age of fifty, post her menopause. She tried everything—diet, tryptophan supplements and homeopathy—but nothing worked because she would eventually grow immune to it. The headaches would get so bad that she would always need medication. An MRI scan showed that everything was normal and finally, her doctor recommended coffee before sleeping at night (weird, as I always thought coffee made things worse). Of late, she gets them in the late evening, instead of in the middle of her sleep-cycle. The case forced me to research some more and then I came across hypnic headaches. These are more common in women than men in a ratio of 9:1. It is believed to be a disorder of the elderly; many people suffer with it for years before they are diagnosed. Most people think it's a migraine.

Shonali Sabherwal

Why Do Migraines Occur?

Migraines are chronic headaches characterized by throbbing pain in response to certain triggers. They are usually preceded by premonitory symptoms which predict the onset. While the exact cause is unknown, migraines may be caused by increase in neurotransmitters, which then cause vasodilatation or swelling of blood vessels.

In the perimenopause, women who have a history of hormone-related menstrual migraine experience a worsening and an increase in the frequency of their headaches. This is believed to be associated with the rise and fall in estrogen and progesterone levels, with these fluctuations increasing significantly in the perimenopause. Besides hormonal changes, migraines may be also triggered by stress, sound and light stimuli and certain foods.

However, for other women, menopause may bring relief and migraine may be replaced by tension headaches. In these women, the use of estrogens in the form of the oral contraceptive pill or MHT might cause a reactivation of the migraine.

What Are the Various Types of Headaches?

Headaches are associated with and manifest because of vasodilatation, although they may have different causes. They may be connected to stress or a change in routine; they have different triggers, many of these coincide with the perimenopause.

- **Sinus Headaches**
  - o Occur due to sinus blockage caused by infection or allergies such as hay fever. Start in the face and there is a stuffy or running nose. Treatment is with decongestants and paracetamol or ibuprofen and nasal, menthol-based products to activate cold receptors.
- **Tension Headaches**
  - o Occur due to physical or emotional stressors triggering the autonomic nervous system. There is a

tight band of pain across the forehead with tightness of neck and shoulders.

- **Cluster Headaches**
  - o Connected to the hypothalamus. They are seasonal, often influenced by light and characterized by a severe, one-sided headache with a running nose.
- **Migraine**
  - o Neurological headache caused by activity in the brain. There is excitation and aura (flashes of light, blind spots and other vision changes or tingling in your hand or face), followed by pain, nausea and sensitivity to light. Estrogen plays a role in occurrence.

Why Do Nighttime Headaches Occur?

Hypnic headaches are nighttime headaches that present in midlife and seem to be connected to the stages of sleep. Genetic inheritance may play a part. An association of a migraine and a variation in the gene for an adenosine receptor could be a link (adenosine, a nucleotide that occurs naturally in the cells, helps in cellular energy transfer and in signalling various pathways and functions in the body). The pain that comes with this type of headache can be a throbbing kind of pain and can be unilateral (occurring on one side) or bilateral (occurring on both sides). Since the headache occurs at night and disrupts sleep, it is called 'alarm-clock' headache.

Hypnic headaches are diagnosed when the following standards are fulfilled:

- They are dull and constant or throbbing.

- They occur during sleep and wake up the person.
- They happen more than fifteen times a month.
- They occur after fifty years of age.
- They have no parallel symptoms such as nausea or blocked sinuses.
- They are not attributable to any other disorder.

The initial approach to headaches, as to VMS, is a modification in lifestyle and diet.

Snapshot on Lifestyle and Diet

Lifestyle Recommendations

- Keep a diary to see what seems to trigger migraines and if they show up along with hot flashes. That way you can take steps to lessen them.
- Do some belly breathing and pranayama.
- Meditate.
- Incorporate exercise and movement.
- Cut back on stress.
- Stay away from bright lights and sunlight.

Diet Recommendations

- Find the food stressors you are intolerant to and eliminate these from your diet.
- Eliminate sugar.
- Eliminate wheat.
- Minimize soy.
- Minimize dairy.
- Minimize caffeine.

When you are a coffee drinker, the blood vessels get constricted. As migraines are caused by enlarged blood vessels in the brain, when you switch off coffee, the vessels remain dilated and you get the migraine. Therefore, have green tea (as it has some caffeine) to keep the blood vessels happy, plus it always helps to keep an ice pack handy.

- Increase the consumption of complex carbohydrates like brown rice and millets as this will not only aid the digestive system, but also help flush out extra unwanted fats in the system.
- Include legumes and lentils in your diet.
- Add chia or flax seeds to your diet for Omega 3 with 1–2 tablespoon a day.

Medical Treatment of Migraine

It is important to recognize the association of perimenopause with headaches and not underplay their significance as being part and parcel of menopause. Headaches at this time may be triggered by hormonal fluctuations or induced by hormone therapy, while in others MHT for VMS may help prevent migraine.

- MHT can worsen headaches in some women, reduce the incidence of headaches in others or cause no changes in yet others. If it worsens your headaches, your estrogen dose may be lowered, changed to a different form of estrogen or stopped.
- An estrogen skin patch or a transdermal gel that provides a low, steady supply of estrogen is least likely to aggravate headaches.

Medicines that help prevent migraines from starting:

- Antidepressants such as amitriptyline and venlafaxine.
- Anticonvulsants such as sodium valproate, valproic acid and topiramate.
- Antihypertensives such as betablockers and calcium-channel blockers.

Medicines that relieve a migraine after it has already started:

- Pain relievers such as paracetamol (acetaminophen), aspirin, ibuprofen and naproxen.
- Triptans such as sumatriptan, rizatriptan, eletriptan and zolmitriptan.
- Botox therapy.

Medical Treatment of Hypnic Headaches

- Caffeine is recommended for hypnic headaches. It is an alkaloid with a natural capacity to constrict blood vessels in the head and neck. Caffeine increases the release of excitatory neurochemicals and so increases the rate of nerve firing. This is why caffeine is stimulating. Caffeine works by blocking adenosine receptors embedded in the surface membranes of nerve cells without activating them, preventing binding to adenosine receptors and blocking its action. This is how caffeine relieves this particular type of headache.
- Lithium and melatonin are also recommended for hypnic headaches.

6

Skin, Hair, Connective Tissues and Cosmetic Changes

'Do not dissect a rainbow. In other words, do not destroy a beautiful phenomenon by overanalyzing it.'

—Denise LaFrance

Most women feel they have started to age in the perimenopause state. A lot of this is psychological, emotional and mental, rather than related to what's actually happening. Vanity often saves the day. We women know that we can affect the way we look, decrease and help prevent wrinkles, sagging skin, lose body fat, maintain muscle mass and increase our energy. We do this by high performance workouts. We get interested and sparked about all the beauty products that would turn it around for us or at least we think they will. So, while the beauty industry will always do well, I get really hassled when women do very little to pay attention to their insides, what they eat and work on their lifestyles to look and feel younger. However, one thing is for sure, the inside, the state of your hormones, your internal organs and overall physiology is what is reflected on the outside.

Shonali Sabherwal

K first consulted me five years ago when she was forty-one years old. She was under treatment for hypothyroidism and hadn't had a period in the last twelve months. She was grappling with hot flushes and irritability, but her greatest concern was the dryness and pigmentation of her skin and accelerated hair loss. Her FSH levels were 60 and estradiol levels were seventeen, suggesting a somewhat early menopause. To give her hormonal protection and balance, I advised her hormone therapy in the form of a fourth-generation, oral contraceptive pill, Drosperinone. This had immediate symptomatic, emotional and cosmetic benefits. I advised her to supplement this with an appropriate diet and vitamin D and E and biotin therapy and regular use of a moisturizer and a higher SPF sun block. A few months later, an antiandrogen finasteride was added to control the hair loss which had persisted. After two years, her only complaint was vaginal dryness and she was switched to conventional MHT with oral conjugated estrogens and progesterone, on which she happily continues to date with periodic monitoring. K loves how she feels and plans to continue MHT until she reaches the age of fifty.

Nozer Sheriar

Your Skin, Your Hair and the Collagen Tissue

With a surface area of 1.5 to 2 square metres, your skin is the largest organ in your body and your interface with the environment that surrounds you. Besides giving you sensory abilities and regulating your temperature, it protects you from infections and manufactures vitamin D. Estrogen receptors are present in the skin cells that produce collagen, which is why with the decrease in estrogen levels after menopause, the body loses collagen and the skin becomes thinner, dryer and less resistant to injury. Collagen is also a major component of the connective tissue that supports your bones and skeletal structure and muscles which are then surrounded by skin.

Estrogen receptors have been detected in many skin elements, including keratinocytes, melanocytes, fibroblasts, hair follicles and sebaceous glands, each with a specialized function. So, it is inevitable that the withdrawal of estrogen at menopause will have significant effects on skin health. After menopause, your skin thins and there is a loss of viscoelasticity. Fortunately, skin-surface texture, water-holding capacity, collagen content of the dermis and elasticity have all shown improvement with the use of estrogen.

Why Does Skin Age?

How we age is also a direct correlation to something called AGEs—advanced glycation end products. AGEs are formed in large amounts in diabetes but are also formed in the process of growing older. Structurally, sugar molecules are either linear or they form a circle, connected at both ends. At a normal pH (that is, when the acid-alkaline balance is maintained), most of the body's glucose is in a circle. This is good for us because a circle is stable. The glucose in linear form is dangerous as it attaches to proteins. This attachment, called cross linking or glycation, results in the formation of AGEs. During menopause, your ability to protect against glycation declines and protein degradation and malfunction become a major cause of ageing.

Now, proteins are the building blocks of life, necessary for many functions in our system and making up much of the body's tissues and organs besides regulating cells, their functions and structures. At the point where sugar attaches to protein, there is a mechanism creating inflammation. When these sugar molecules attach to the collagen protein, wrinkles are formed as the inflammation produces enzymes that break down collagen. AGEs are kicked into motion by consuming sugar, refined carbohydrates, high-glycaemic foods and throwing the normal insulin response off.

Hormones have a lot to do with skin as well. Progesterone, estrogen and testosterone maintain the normal balance called homeostasis. In the perimenopause, the declining estrogen levels speed up the process of skin ageing. This leads to a decrease in skin collagen with a breakdown in structure and promotes the appearance of wrinkles. The skin loses elasticity, mobility, turgidity and fluid content.

Besides this, there is a loss of melanocytes, the cells which produce the pigment called melanin that protect you from sunlight. This makes your skin photosensitive and prone to sunburn and collagen destruction with patches of brown pigmentation and freckles. There is also a decreased vascularity and a decline in the activity of the sebaceous glands that leads to reduced lubrication, dryness and flaking.

Why Is There Increased Hair Fall?

The decrease in estrogen levels affects the health and growth of hair. Estrogen receptors in the hair follicles maintain the growth cycle and the normal pattern of female hair distribution. From the perimenopause, hair begins to lose its texture, body and thickness and becomes thinner, finer and weaker. The collagen deficiency also leads to poor growth, split ends, hair loss and flaking and dermatitis of the scalp.

As one is in the anovulation mode during the perimenopause, hair fall is a common complaint. Most women witness a strange pattern of balding above their temples in the frontal left and right side of the head around this time. When progesterone falls, the body responds by the increase of the adrenal cortical steroid, androstenedione, an alternative precursor for the production of the adrenal cortical hormones and testosterone. Moreover, high androgens are usually accompanied by high DHT levels. Both androstenedione and DHT cause male pattern of baldness.

Why Do Some Women Experience Hair Loss?

Female pattern hair loss (FPHL) is also referred to as androgenetic alopecia. The commonest cause of hair loss in women, it presents as progressive hair thinning at the vertex of the scalp with sparing of the frontal hairline. It most commonly begins at or soon after menopause and can cause significant psychological distress. Although the role of androgens and genetic susceptibility is recognized in male-pattern hair loss, it is less well understood in FPHL, with the majority of women with FPHL having no features or evidence of excess androgens.

Why Is There Increased Facial Hair?

Hirsutism is a condition in women that results in excessive hair growth, in a male-like pattern. In hirsutism, stiff or dark hair appear on the body where women don't commonly have hair, primarily the face, chest, lower abdomen, inner thighs and back. There are widely varying opinions on what growth is considered excessive. To standardize diagnosis, doctors use the Ferriman-Gallwey scale, where a score of one to four is given for nine areas of the body. A total score less than eight is considered normal, a score of eight to fifteen indicates mild hirsutism and a score greater than fifteen indicates moderate or severe hirsutism.

Hirsutism is caused by a dominance of the androgens, generally testosterone centrally and DHT locally. In perimenopause, along with the fall in estrogen levels, there develops an imbalance with androgens, the male hormones that are also present in women. This increase in the androgen to estrogen ratio results in a conversion of

Figure 6: Scale for excess male-pattern hair growth

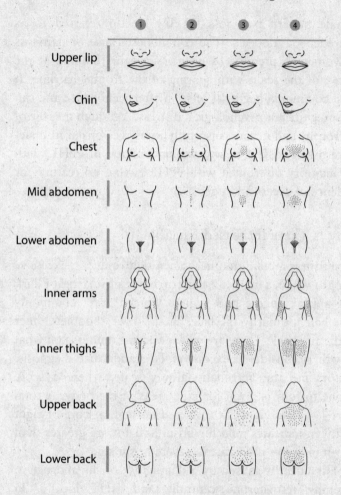

Adapted from the The Ferriman-Gallwey scale for excess male-pattern hair growth

the fine, unpigmented hair on the upper lip, chin, chest and axillary and pubic region to thicker and darker hair.

Estrogen therapy may help address the falling levels of estrogen that lead to androgen dominance and cause hirsutism. Anti-androgen therapy may be required in some cases. Medications such as anabolic steroids, minoxidil and phenytoin may also be a cause.

Why Do Muscles and Joints Ache?

Generalized muscle and joint aches are among the commonest symptoms experienced by women at menopause. While the effects of estrogen on bone are well known, studies on the impact of estrogen deficiency on cartilage and connective tissues have been slower to emerge. Recent studies have identified estrogen receptors in chondrocytes (cells producing cartilage matrix) and synoviocytes (cells producing the synovial fluid responsible for joint lubrication). Although no clear association has been found between estrogen exposure and the risk of osteoarthritis, the marked predominance of osteoarthritis in women and, in particular, the marked increase after menopause suggests that female sex steroids are important for health of cartilage. Arthritis in women is more likely to be progressive and symptomatic. Research has demonstrated protective effects on cartilage and joints from the use of estrogen and a 45 per cent reduction in total joint surgery among women taking MHT.

Fortunately, most of these changes, although they may be distressing, can be countered by diet, lifestyle modifications and medical treatment.

Snapshot on Lifestyle and Diet

Lifestyle Recommendations

- Exercise, including cardio and strength. Pilates, yoga, weight training or functional are all good options.
- Be regular with mealtimes.
- Regulate sleep habits.
- Keep stress under control. Excessive cortisol due to stress will aggravate inflammation, which will harm the skin and resulting in sugar cravings, which is the worst situation to be in for skin health.
- Many skincare products contain endocrine-disrupting chemicals (EDCs). These interfere with hormone function and get absorbed into the skin, causing problems. So, know the products you are using. Some things to watch out for are parabens, oxybenzone (sunscreens) and products that have perfume.
- Practise meditation and pranayama. Nothing like being calm for good skin.
- Keep digestive distress to a minimum.
- Stop smoking, even avoiding second-hand smoke.
- Minimize exposure to the sun.

Diet Recommendations

Skin, hair and cosmetic issues get aggravated by the foods you eat, as foods have their own energy and ways of elimination. The only place your blood condition, whether imbalanced or balanced, shows up is in the outward body—the skin, hair and nails. With skin, hair and nails, I seek to balance the blood condition to make it less acidic in nature and strengthen the gut. All the dietary recommendations below stem from eliminating or minimizing foods that cause an aggravation of the condition itself, that is, removing pro-inflammatory foods.

Inflammation is recognized as a problem affecting muscles and joints. Macrobiotic philosophy focuses on eating certain kinds of food impacting different parts of the body. This is also explained in the diet section of the book:

- Avoid sugars, including hidden sugars in products.
- Watch out for high glycaemic index (GI) foods and eat low GI foods. Foods high in sugar trigger the insulin response, leading to the aggravation of AGEs which weaken protein and cause collagen damage. Also, sugars lead to an acidic blood condition and weaken kidney energy, causing the hair quality to deteriorate.
- Minimize dairy and dairy products since an overuse of dairy leads to acidic blood condition, causing hair and skin quality to deteriorate. Plus, dairy makes you crave more sugar.
- Exclude foods with additives and food colours since you don't need something coming in that is not processed by the body well.
- Avoid artificial sweeteners since they throw off your insulin response.
- Avoid hydrogenated fats, trans fats and refined oils, as there is a lot of free radical damage that happens with these fats.
- Avoid monosodium glutamate (MSG) since it has been connected to skin eruptions.
- Coffee, sodas and colas do not help with their added sugars.

- Occasional consumption of fried foods, with the right oils, is all right. However, excessive fried foods in your diet will cause free radical damage and lead to an increase in inflammation.
- Alcohol has empty sugars and will trigger your insulin response, also causing inflammation if overdone.
- Minimize xenoestrogen exposure (discussed in the diet section) since they will throw your hormones off.
- Include high-fibre foods, as you need fibre to clear excess testosterone.
- Eat foods that have zinc, such as sesame seeds, pumpkin seeds, tofu, tempeh, edamame, hemp seeds, cashews, pine nuts, lentils, shiitake mushrooms, spinach and green peas.
- Good quality protein will keep the collagen and keratin strong for skin and hair.
- Add fermented foods, as there is a strong connection between your gut and skin, hair and the manifestations of beauty. Strengthening the diverse strains of good bacteria in your gut will not only help your gut, but also impact all your organs and immunity.
- Add garlic, even if using an extract. It is an antioxidant with multiple benefits.
- Use cinnamon (½ teaspoon in water daily) to bring down insulin levels.

Include a supplement with a blend of mushrooms, maitake, shiitake and cordyceps, to help with blood condition and aid in detoxification of harmful xenoestrogens.

- Adding a collagen supplement or bone broth to your diet really helps.

- A supplement with a blend of mushrooms: maitake, shiitake and cordyceps.

Medical Management

The skin and connective tissues go through significant changes during the perimenopause. This is in part due to the changes in hormone levels and in part because of the preceding years of damage and neglect. If you have spent ample time in the sun without sun protection, you will likely see the effects now. Age spots and larger areas of darker skin can appear on your face, hands, neck, arms, or chest. However, it is never too late to start. The care of skin and connective tissues needs a multispecialty team which includes a gynaecologist, an endocrinologist, a dietician, a dermatologist and a cosmetologist.

Skincare Supplements to Use

- Alpha lipoic acid (ALA) counteracts the effects of ageing, thwarts inflammation, produces free radicals and boosts glutathione, which is critical for an optimum immune system.
- Omega 3 essential fatty acids, including foods like oily fish, chia and flax seeds, protects against sun damage, reduces itchy skin and helps with skin repair.
- Co Q10 is a key antioxidant for mitochondrial support, rejuvenation and repair. It is found in foods but supplementing it at this time really helps.
- Glutathione helps cells to detoxify and protects them against the processes of AGEs.

- Resveratrol is part of a group of compounds called polyphenols. They act like antioxidants, protecting the body against damage by helping to fight AGEs.
- Hyaluronic acid helps reduce fine lines, keeps skin extra hydrated.

Skincare Medical Essentials

- For age spots and to reduce the risk of cancer, apply sunscreen every day before going outdoors.
  - o Use a sunscreen with SPF 30 or higher and apply it to all exposed skin. Sunscreen also benefits thin skin that bruises easily. While it cannot thicken your skin, it can prevent further thinning.
  - o A retinoid cream and laser treatment following a dermatologist consultation may be other options to reduce age spots.
- For dry skin, wash with a mild cleanser instead of soap since soap can be too drying for mature skin. You definitely want to skip the deodorant bars. Application of a moisturizer with hyaluronic acid or glycerine after bathing can be especially helpful. Your dermatologist could help you with exfoliation or microdermabrasion.
- For jowls, slack skin and wrinkles resulting from collagen loss, protect your skin from the sun to reduce visible wrinkles and prevent new wrinkles. Skincare products containing retinol or peptides can increase collagen in your skin.
- For pimples and other types of acne, treatments for teenage acne are often too harsh. Instead, wash acne-prone skin with a cleanser that contains salicylic acid,

which helps unclog pores, and avoid products that dry your skin. If you cannot get acne under control, hormonal treatment may be necessary.

- During perimenopause, the pH level of your skin changes, with skin becoming more sensitive and prone to develop rashes and irritation. Existing skin conditions such as eczema or rosacea could worsen. Use a fragrance-free moisturizer to reduce irritation and seek the help of a dermatologist if symptoms persist or worsen.

- Estrogen therapy has been shown to diminish skin ageing with an increased dermal thickness resulting in increased skin thickness. It also increases the collagen content of the skin, decreasing facial wrinkling this being considered a collateral benefit of long-term MHT.

Haircare Supplements to Use

- Add chromium (200 to 1000 mcg) per day as an insulin sensitizer.
- Add inositol to improve insulin sensitivity.
- Add a vitamin D supplement.

Haircare Medical Essentials

- Physical modalities are the first line treatment for hirsutism. Excessive facial hair, the unwanted hair under your chin, along your jawline or above your lip can be concealed by bleaching or removed by waxing or electrolysis. Laser hair removal following hormone therapy gives the best results.
- During perimenopause, low dose COCs are found to be effective to suppress hirsutism.

- For moderate to severe hirsutism, particularly with elevated testosterone or DHT levels, antiandrogens that counter the elevated male hormones are to be used under specialist care. Spironolactone is the first-line therapy. Finasteride and cyproterone are second-line antiandrogens. Flutamide is highly effective with elevated DHT but its use needs careful monitoring of liver function.
- For hair loss on your head, which generally starts as a widening of the parting followed by a receding hairline, the earlier you start treatment the better the results. For considerable hair loss, a hair transplant may become a necessity.
- The use of topical minoxidil available as a 2 per cent lotion and a 5 per cent lotion or foam is the only licensed treatment for FPHL.

Magical Treatment for Hair Growth

Use Indralupta Lepam (source available at soulfoodshonali. com)

- Grate 2–3 shallots.
- Squeeze juice and apply with cotton wool to affected parts of the scalp.
- Remove a small amount of indralupata lepam and apply on bald areas.
- Leave for 30 minutes and then wash off.
- Repeat thrice a week, or daily if you are losing a lot of hair.

7

Vaginal and Urogenital Changes and Disturbance

'As our body journeys through life and life journeys on our body . . . life will leave marks on us too.'

—Lauren Klarfeld

Recently, Doc insisted I go for all my tests. We were still working on the book, and this was post the COVID lockdown. Technically, I had already skipped a year of annual examination. His assistant doctor conducted the pap smear. Before I go forward with this story, let me tell you that my threshold of physical pain is very high. But when she put the speculum into me, I shrieked with pain. I was in shock, so I started clenching my butt, which only made it worse. She kept encouraging me to release my butt and ease out, but I was frozen.

'Don't you feel the pain when you are having sex?' she asked me.

And in the middle of that pain, I retorted, 'What makes you assume I'm having any sex!'

We both laughed a bit, and then she said, 'I'm so sorry, but you're extremely dry and that's why it's hurting.'

I had no mental map of the insides of my vagina. Not having been sexually active for a while and being perimenopausal, how would I have known?

In a conversation later with Dr Nozer, I said, 'I was amazed to see that someone like me, who takes care of myself on the food front, the exercise front and the mental front could go through vaginal atrophy.'

His answer to me was, 'You can't beat nature.' Not being sexually active could have put me in this situation sooner, but there is a way out—the current estrogen cream I am using is really helping. I first contemplated not using it, but Dr Nozer told me that I should, as he did not want further changes taking place. Besides, I am hopeful of yet again being in a relationship where this condition will not pose an issue.

Shonali Sabherwal

I first met K fifteen years ago when she was forty-five years old and menopausal for the past year. She complained of being bloated and tired, of frequent urination and vaginal dryness and swelling. She was *on isoflavones for two years with limited relief. I initially treated with oral estriol and then tibolone, off and on for eight years. Since then, her only complaint has been vaginal dryness and atrophy, for which I have prescribed vaginal estrogens, either conjugated estrogen or estriol. She has benefited greatly from the estrogen creams but for some reason she has found it difficult, almost impossible, to use the applicator for intravaginal application. She has worked out that a fortnightly or even monthly application combined with her use of homeopathy seems to work well for her. For many years now, she visits the clinic once or twice a month to have the vaginal estrogen application done by us and to tell us how well she is doing. K has shown me once more that women know best what works for them, even though it may not seem very scientific to the doctor. We shouldn't just hear them, we need to listen to them.*

Nozer Sheriar

The Vagina, Pelvic Organs and Pelvic Floor

Your vagina and the pelvic structures are rich in estrogen receptors. With a decrease in estrogen levels, the vagina begins to atrophy and the lining tends to become dry and thinned out. With a decrease in the activity of the vaginal glands the mucus secretion reduces, making the vagina less lubricated and more prone to abrasions and infections. These changes in the vagina are accompanied by a thinning and shrinkage of the tissues of the vulva, urethra and bladder.

This results in multiple symptoms such as vaginal dryness, vaginal irritation, a frequent need to urinate and urinary tract infections. There are also changes in the opening of the vagina, the vulva. The vaginal labial lips become thin and flat and the perineum, the area just behind the vaginal opening, becomes thinner and dryer making it prone to itching and bruising or abrasion with slow healing.

The muscles of the floor of the pelvis form a diaphragm that supports the pelvic organs, the uterus, bladder and the rectum. Estrogen plays an important role in maintaining this support system, which counters the effects of gravity and increased abdominal pressure. Women do have a distinct disadvantage compared with men in that the vaginal opening leaves a potential point of weakness if the pelvic floor develops laxity. With decreasing estrogen levels, menopause leads to a loss of tone and elasticity, leading to sagging of the vaginal walls, descent of the uterus and pelvic organ prolapse.

Since the urinary tract is right next to the vagina, urinary complaints often manifest during the perimenopause. Some women experience urge incontinence, which is a feeling of urgency, difficulty, loss of control and leakage due to an irritable bladder. Others experience stress incontinence, which is a leakage of urine when they cough, sneeze or strain, due to a weakness or a loss of tone of the muscle supporting the bladder.

A study of menopausal Indian women reported urogenital symptoms in 15 per cent, with vaginal dryness in 32 per cent, itching in 15 per cent and painful sex and urinary urgency in 10 per cent. Most women suffer these complaints in silence, assuming these to be normal. You should not. You must seek out medical help early to prevent worsening of these conditions.

The following diagram shows the distribution of estrogen receptors in the pelvis. They are found to be concentrated in the vagina and uterus, their supports and muscles of the pelvic floor, the lower bladder wall and the urethra.

Figure 7: Distribution of estrogen receptors in the pelvic structures

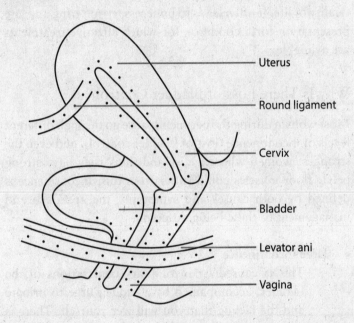

- Uterus
- Round ligament
- Cervix
- Bladder
- Levator ani
- Vagina

Why Is There Vaginal Dryness?

After menopause, structural and functional changes in the vagina and urogenital lining (epithelium) appear due to a drop in estrogen levels. More than half of all post-menopausal women will experience symptoms associated with tissue atrophy.

The term genitourinary syndrome of menopause (GSM) has been proposed as an alternative to vulvovaginal atrophy (VVA), to describe more accurately the constellation of urogenital complaints and signs associated with menopause and to remove the negative connotation of the term atrophy.

Many women lack awareness that GSM is a chronic condition with a significant impact on sexual health and quality of life. It often leads to unnecessary suffering and late presentation for a condition for which effective treatments are available.

Why Is There Loss of Bladder Control?

Most women during the perimenopause go through different levels of incontinence (loss of bladder control), and even the strongest women who exercise and think they have strong pelvic floor muscles could suffer from this. Incontinence is defined by both causes and symptoms, the approach and management to these being different:

- Urge incontinence
    - This is caused by involuntary contractions of the bladder, accompanied by a sudden urge to urinate and the feeling that you will wet yourself. There is often urgency and loss of control when changing position, say when standing from a sitting position or just as you reach the rest room. Usually caused by overreactive and irritated bladder muscles, urge incontinence also has a strong involuntary component. The bladder irritation could occur due to localized lack of estrogen in the bladder and urethral area, which is also associated with

perimenopause and menopause. In rare cases, the urgency of bladder incontinence may be compounded by rectal urgency and incontinence.

Figure 8: Mechanism of urge incontinence

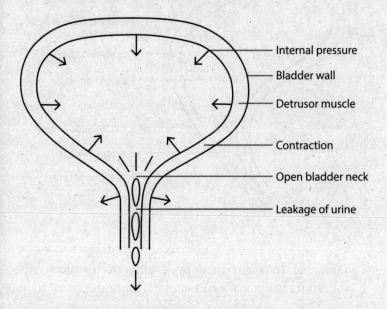

- Stress incontinence
  o This is caused by a weak pelvic floor. Your bladder might leak if you sneeze, cough, laugh, lift a heavy object or stress—anything that causes a sudden increase in abdominal pressures. It is a common pre-menopausal symptom and does not generally worsen during menopause.

Figure 9: Mechanism of stress urinary incontinence

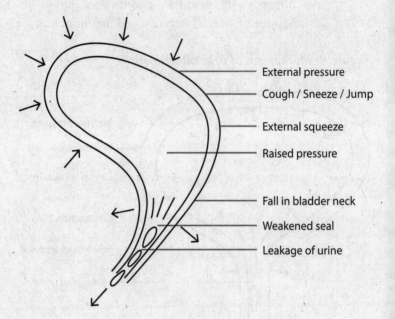

External pressure

Cough / Sneeze / Jump

External squeeze

Raised pressure

Fall in bladder neck

Weakened seal

Leakage of urine

Urodynamic tests are used by doctors to confirm and quantify urinary incontinence and diagnose the type. They measure nerve and muscle function, the pressure around and in the bladder, flow rates and other factors and look at how well the bladder, the sphincter and the urethra are storing and releasing urine.

Incontinence is not a natural phenomenon of ageing, and you must take it up seriously if it starts happening. You will need to train your pelvic floor and there is a section at the end of this book that addresses this. For severe incontinence, medical or surgical treatment may be needed.

Why Do Pelvic Organs Prolapse?

The organs within a woman's pelvis—her uterus, bladder and rectum—are normally held in place by ligaments and muscles known as the pelvic floor. If these are weakened, the pelvic organs can be displaced from their natural position into the vagina. This is known as pelvic organ prolapse. While prolapse is not considered a life-threatening condition and some women can have a prolapse without having any symptoms at all, it may cause a great deal of discomfort and distress.

Common symptoms of prolapse include:

- A feeling of dragging or heaviness in the pelvic area.
- A bulge in the front or back wall of the vagina, sometimes this bulging extending outside the vagina.
- Difficulties with continence, bladder or bowel, depending on the location of the prolapse.
  - Prolapse of the bladder may cause frequency, hesitancy and a feeling of incomplete emptying.
  - Prolapse of the rectum may cause constipation, discomfort and a feeling of incomplete evacuation.
- Discomfort and a lack of sensation during sex.

Prolapse may be uterine prolapse, where the uterus comes down from its position; or vaginal prolapse, where there is a bulging of the anterior vaginal wall along with the bladder (cystocele) or the posterior vaginal wall along with the rectum (rectocele), although it is generally a combination of both. The stretching of the supports of the uterus and the pelvic floor usually happens during childbirth but it is with the decrease in estrogen levels and the loss of muscle

Figure 10: Types of pelvic organ prolapse

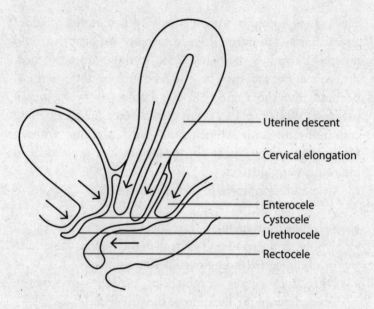

Uterine descent

Cervical elongation

Enterocele
Cystocele
Urethrocele
Rectocele

and ligament tone that the prolapse presents and causes discomfort and symptoms after menopause.

Why Do Urinary Infections Occur?

A urinary tract infection (UTI) is an infection that occurs in any part of your urinary system, including your urethra, bladder, ureters and kidneys. As estrogen production falls in menopausal women, UTIs can occur more frequently. There are several reasons for this. During the perimenopause your vaginal tissue thins, making it more prone to infection. Women may also have trouble fully emptying the bladder due to a vaginal prolapse, which can increase the chance of an infection due to the stagnant pool of urine. With less estrogen in your body, bacterial levels can change, allowing infection to set in. Some menopausal women have occasional, acute UTIs, but others experience chronic, frustrating UTIs that occur month after month after month and interfere with their quality of life and, by extension, sexual enjoyment.

Why Do Vaginal Infections Occur?

Decreased estrogen and progesterone in post-menopausal women make vaginal tissues thinner and less elastic. These vaginal atrophic changes affect up to half of all post-menopausal women, and lead to changes in vaginal pH, cellular glycogen content and vaginal microflora, all of which play roles in vulvovaginal symptoms such as vaginal infections. Women with vaginal infections report a number of vaginal complaints, such as external and internal itching, pain, irritation, soreness, urinary burning, abnormal vaginal discharge and painful sex.

The most frequent infections are bacterial vaginosis (BV) and vulvovaginal candidiasis (VVC). Since BV occurs under more alkaline vaginal conditions (pH > 4.5) due to colonization by anaerobic (low-oxygen environment) bacteria and fewer lactobacilli (the good bacteria in the vagina), it is more frequent in post-menopausal women who have low glycogen and vaginal pH >5. Since vaginal pH tends to be lowered by hormone therapy, VVC tends to dominate in this situation.

Snapshot on Lifestyle and Diet

Lifestyle Recommendations

- Use a douche made with two cups apple cider vinegar diluted with four cups of water and use it twice a day.

This helps remove any harmful accumulation of toxins in the vaginal area and balances pH. Douching is done using a douche spray bulb.

- Do a Sitz bath by boiling either dried radish leaves or arame (seaweed) in 2 litres of water for about twenty minutes. Strain the water and add to a tub till it reaches your waist. Sit in the tub once daily for twenty minutes. This is a useful home remedy to flush out any inflammation, pain, swelling or irritation in the perineum and also flush out toxins and promote blood flow. It also helps get rid of mucous and stagnation in the reproductive areas. However, both douching and Sitz bath should be avoided if their use causes local vulvar or vaginal irritation.
- Do not wear tight underwear and use cotton at all times. This helps the vagina breathe.
- Do not use powders in the vaginal area as these can have unwanted irritants and there is some evidence of linkage with ovarian cancer.
- Include Kegel exercises (see the section on exercise).
- Add pranayama (breathing) to bring in oxygen to the cells of our body and ameliorate everything that's going wrong in all areas of the body.
- Exercise to release endorphins (feel-good hormones) and focus less on the discomfort bought about by changes during this time.

Diet Recommendations

Detailed guidance and explanations are provided in the diet section. Vaginal and urogenital systems get aggravated by the foods you eat, as foods have their own energy. All the dietary recommendations below are based on eliminating or minimizing foods that would cause an aggravation of the condition itself, that is removing pro-inflammatory foods. Inflammation has become a huge problem, underlying almost all conditions.

A breakdown of gut bacteria is another element at play here, since dysbiosis will cause issues like growth of negative bacteria and fungi like candida albicans. All foods listed below will address this breakdown of the inner ecosystem. Macrobiotic philosophy focuses on the fact that eating too many foods of one nature causes you to try and compensate by craving foods of the opposite nature. I have also explained this in the diet section of the book.

- Minimize consumption of alcohol and caffeinated drinks. These will increase acidic blood condition and dehydrate you. Alcohol is avoidable due to empty sugars and yeast in foods or drinks as well at this time.
- Minimize eating dairy, as it does not get totally absorbed by the body and the residue tends to cause the blood to get acidic and adds to the mucous in the body.
- Quit sugar, including refined white flour (maida) or products off the shelf that have hidden sugars. Sugar plays havoc on the system. It causes acidic blood condition, robs you of gut bacteria and is what we call a 'yin food' causing your body to have a mind of its own as soon as you consume it.
- Minimize fruit juices, although fruit is fine. Having fruit juices where more than one fruit is used to make the juice is too much fructose for the body to handle and the body treats it as it would sugar.
- Quit packaged foods as you don't really know what could cause an imbalance in vaginal pH and also a breakdown of gut and vaginal 'good' bacteria.

- Increase the consumption of fibre like brown rice and millets, lentils, nuts and seeds and fruits as these will not only aid the digestive system in elimination due to their high-fibre content, but will also keep your sugars steady bringing in the balance you need and help feed gut and vaginal bacteria.
- Use turmeric as it is an anti-inflammatory. It will help control all the other negatives that come in when eating goes haywire during this time but use it in moderation. The way we Indians use it as a part of our Indian cooking is adequate.

Medical Management

Genitourinary Syndrome of Menopause (GSM)

Vaginal Estrogen Therapy

Vaginal therapy in the form of local application of estrogen creams is most effective in the treatment of urogenital dryness and atrophy and is as effective as systemic therapy. In fact, some women on oral estrogens may require additional local therapy if the vaginal response is inadequate. The estrogen cream is to be applied in the vagina with a metered applicator (not with a finger) twice or thrice a week. Progesterone supplement for endometrial protection is not needed along with the use of vaginal estrogen and regular endometrial check up by ultrasound is not necessary. Vaginal estrogen can safely be used by women in whom systemic HRT is contraindicated.

If vaginal estrogen does not relieve the symptoms of urogenital atrophy, the dose or frequency of use can be increased. It is important to remember that with urogenital atrophy, symptoms often come back when treatment is stopped and hence the treatment should be long term. Treatment should be started early to prevent irreversible atrophic changes and continued long term to maintain benefits. After control of acute symptoms, the dose of local estrogen can be tapered for maintenance therapy and treatment may be continued indefinitely. All local estrogen preparations (creams, pessaries, tablets, vaginal ring) are effective in decreasing signs and symptoms of vaginal atrophy. Repeated vaginal and urinary tract infections will also benefit from the local estrogen application with simultaneous local or systemic treatment of the infections.

Since there is limited data on the use of vaginal estrogens in women with breast cancer, lifestyle management and nonhormonal treatments would be the first option. However, in resistant cases, in joint consultation with the oncologist, vaginal estrogen may be used with a low-potency agent like estriol.

Non-Hormonal Options

GSM is a chronic condition with a significant impact on sexual health and quality of life. Vaginal moisturizers and lubricants play an important role in relieving symptoms of painful sex. Vaginal moisturizers have an equivalent efficacy to topical vaginal estrogen and should be offered to women wishing to avoid the use of hormonal therapy.

There is evidence that regular sexual activity maintains vaginal health and since local estrogens and the use of moisturizers and lubricants counteract dryness and pain and make sexual activity pleasant for the woman, they, in turn, have a definite role in improving long-term, vaginal health.

Diet Recommendations

- Drink corn silk tea which is packed with minerals and antioxidants.
  - o Take a tablespoon of chopped corn silk and 1 cup of water. Boil for 15–20 minutes and drink after straining.
  - o It can be stored in the refrigerator for up to three days.
- Add a magnesium supplement or magnesium-rich foods like bananas, almonds, sunflower seeds and broccoli to your diet.
- Increase vitamin D intake from fish, eggs and by supplementation.

Management of Urinary Incontinence

Urge Incontinence

Lifestyle changes and bladder training have been shown to be effective for overactive bladder symptoms and are first-line therapy.

- **Bladder training,** where you start by trying to hold your urine for five minutes every time you feel the urge to urinate. Gradually increase the time to ten minutes. Continue to increase the time until you are urinating every three to four hours. When you feel the urge to urinate before your time is up, you can try relaxation techniques by breathing slow and deep until the urge goes away. Kegel exercises may also help. It may take one to three months of training to show results, so please persist.

- **Vaginal estrogen** administration supplements the behavioural treatment of urge incontinence.
- **Bladder-relaxing drugs** such as tolterodine, solifenacin and mirabegron that relax and quieten the bladder muscle, combined with local estrogens, constitute second-line medical treatment in post-menopausal women with an overactive bladder.

Stress Urinary Incontinence (SUI)

Women complaining of stress urinary incontinence will benefit from pelvic floor muscle training in the first instance.

- **Bladder-control products** are dedicated products available over the counter or online. They include incontinence pads, disposable underwear and linen to catch any leak and pull moisture away from your skin. Many are designed to block odour and have a waterproof backing to prevent the overflow from reaching your clothes.
- **Kegel exercises**, where you contract your pelvic floor and pretend you are trying to stop urinary flow. Pull in and squeeze those muscles. Hold the squeeze for about ten seconds and then rest for ten seconds. Try to do three to four sets of ten contractions every day; you can do these exercises at any time and anywhere. It may take three to six weeks of exercise to show results so please persist. There are also devices such as vaginal weights or

cones that you may use to assist in the exercises. Once you see benefits, please continue with the exercises. It is never too early or too late to start this exercise.

- **Duloxetine** may sometimes work in combination with conservative therapy.
- **SUI surgery** for women with frank SUI, to create a fresh support for the bladder neck using a synthetic tape, is the best option. The procedure of placing the trans-obturator tape is now standardized and is a minimally invasive procedure. This is combined with a vaginal repair if that is considered clinically essential. There are alternative procedures such as a Burch colposuspension but these are rarely performed.

Management of Pelvic Organ Prolapse

The treatment of pelvic organ prolapse depends on the type, the extent and the severity of complaints. Some degree of pelvic organ prolapse is present in most women after vaginal birth; some degree of pelvic organ prolapse is caused by the weakening of the supports of the uterus and the vagina at menopause. Prolapse being a structural problem, the only effective treatment for significant prolapse is surgical repair. However, surgery must be avoided if there are no significant symptoms and not be conducted willy-nilly just because an examination finds some descent.

Treatment of pelvic organ prolapse can include a variety of therapies:

- **Behavioural treatments** such as physical therapy to strengthen the muscles of your core and Kegel exercises to maintain the pelvic floor muscles in good tone.

- **Mechanical treatments** using a small plastic device called a ring pessary in the vagina to provide support for the drooping organs. This treatment is for lower degrees of severity and short-term use in women who are not ready for or at high risk for surgical treatment.
- **Vaginal estrogen therapy** will not help existing prolapse but is used before surgery to make the vagina healthier.
- **Surgical treatment,** either to repair the affected tissue or to remove the prolapsed uterus.
  o Vaginal repair of the anterior vaginal wall (cystocele repair) reduces the prolapse and strengthens the fascia supporting the bladder wall.
  o Vaginal repair of the posterior vaginal wall (rectocele repair) reduces the prolapse and strengthens the fascia supporting the rectal wall.
  o Hysterectomy surgically removes the uterus through the vaginal route where there is significant descent of the uterus. Vaginal hysterectomy and vaginal repairs are invariably combined in the same procedure and are the most frequent surgeries performed for perimenopausal prolapse.
  o Conservative surgeries such as vaginal and abdominal slings are an option in younger women where the uterus needs to be retained.

Female Genital Cosmetic Surgery and Vaginal Rejuvenation

Female genital cosmetic surgery (FGCS) includes procedures performed either for aesthetic reasons or to improve sexual functioning. They include vaginal rejuvenation to increase vaginal tone, labiaplasty to trim and reduce the size of the labia minora, vulvar liposculpturing for the labia major and G-spot amplification using hyaluronic acid injection. Much vaginal rejuvenation involves procedures performed to decrease the average diameter of the vagina, mainly for sexual reasons. These procedures are meant to correct problems such as vaginal laxity, stress incontinence or lack of lubrication that can occur after childbirth or during the ageing process.

There are two types of energy-based treatments for vaginal rejuvenation. Both types of treatment use heat to heat up the top layers of the vaginal tissue so that the underlying layers create extra collagen to help heal the area and make new and firmer tissue.

- Radiofrequency (RF) treatments where electromagnetic waves focus energy to heat the tissue.
- Laser treatment where the CO2 laser heats up the upper layers of the tissue.

Many professional medical organizations have released statements discouraging female genital cosmetic procedures which do not include medically indicated reconstructions. Gynaecological conditions that merit surgery include genital prolapse, SUI repairs, reconstructive surgery following female genital mutilation and labiaplasties for medical indications. The performance of cosmetic procedures for indications other than these currently lacks scientific evidence of effectiveness and safety, with risk of complications such as scarring, adhesions, infection and painful sex and altered sexual sensation.

Recurrent Urinary Tract Infections

Sometimes urge incontinence could be the result of a urinary tract infection. Here, your gynaecologist can examine you to check the outer urethra and if it is not estrogenized, reddened and thinned out, prescribe an estrogen cream.

The female genital and lower urinary tracts share a common developmental (embryological) origin, arising from a common urogenital sinus, so both are sensitive to the effects of female hormones throughout life. Estrogen is known to have an important role in the function of the lower urinary tract and estrogen and progesterone receptors have been demonstrated in the vagina, urethra, bladder and pelvic floor musculature. Consequently, exogenous estrogen therapy may be useful in the management of pelvic floor dysfunction and recurrent UTI. Its use in urogenital atrophy and UTI correlates with symptom relief by improving vaginal dryness, itching, improving cytological findings and response to antibiotic treatment of UTI.

Management of Recurrent Urinary Tract Infections

Estrogen therapy has been shown to decrease vaginal pH and reverse the microbiological changes that occur in the vagina following menopause and has been shown to be useful in the prevention of recurrent UTIs. Urogenital symptoms respond well to estrogens. Long-term treatment is often required as symptoms can recur upon cessation of therapy. Local, low-potency, low-dose estrogens in the form of creams or gels used with an applicator twice or thrice a week are effective and safe with no systemic risks or side effects. In the face of these, systemic MHT does not seem to be preferable to low dose local estrogens in the management of atrophy or recurrent lower urinary tract infections.

Simultaneous treatment of mixed infections by local antibiotic and anti-fungal vaginal pessaries as also oral medications could be needed since there is often an association between urinary and vaginal infections.

- Where possible, the organism causing the infection should be identified by doing a urine culture, which will also help with selecting effective antibiotics that the infection will be sensitive to.
  o Single-dose fosfomycin could be used for immediate relief.
  o Choice of antibiotic is dictated by the culture sensitivity report. Ciprofloxacin, ofloxacin, cephalosporins and nitrofurantoin are the commonly used antibiotics and the dose and duration advised by the doctor should be strictly adhered to.
  o Self-medication or inadequate and incomplete courses of treatment should be avoided as these will lead to resistant infections in the long run.
- The importance of adequate fluid intake cannot be overstressed.
- The use of urinary alkalizers, cranberry juice or extract and D-mannose alleviates symptoms and protects against infection.
- Probiotics with 'good' bacteria used as adjunctive therapy would ensure vaginal health and protect against recurrence.

Management of Recurrent Vaginal Infections

My own history with yeast infections is a story that can be a whole new book for women. These infections are characterized by the overgrowth of candida albicans, the bacteria found in the gastrointestinal tract, vaginal pathways, mouth and skin, and wherever they get a warm and moist anaerobic (without oxygen) environment. Over 80 per cent of women suffer from these at some point in their life. Symptoms could be vaginal itching, redness, thick cheese-like discharge and recurrent UTIs.

In a healthy vaginal space, the normal bacteria— lactobacilli—dominate and drown out candida albicans. Many things could lead to an overgrowth of candida—a bad diet full of sugar, empty carbohydrates and junk food (basically anything to do with sugar); antibiotic treatment for other infections; stress or over-douching, which could disturb your vaginal pH. Higher estrogen levels cause a rise in glucose in vaginal mucosa, leading to the growth of candida. It is imperative to have normal levels of both estrogen and progesterone to inhibit the growth of candida and it took me seven years of the 'Hormone-Transformation Diet' to get rid of the bacteria.

Shonali Sabherwal

While there is no direct link between perimenopause and vaginal yeast infections, there may be a modest relationship. A normal, healthy vaginal microflora mainly comprises lactobacilli, which act beneficially as a bacterial barrier in the vagina. Decreased estrogen secretion in post-menopausal women depletes these lactobacilli and increases intravaginal pH, resulting in increased vaginal colonization by harmful microorganisms.

As you get older, there is an increased incidence of diabetes, which could predispose you to yeast infections. Besides this, antibiotic treatment for other infections can change the normal composition of the good protective bacteria in the vagina, the lactobacilli, and this could also lead to yeast infections, so try to avoid taking them unless absolutely necessary.

Three common types of vaginal infections cause vaginitis:

- **Bacterial vaginosis (BV)**
  - This constitutes 40 per cent to 50 per cent of all cases of vaginitis. It usually occurs in vaginal environments that show an increase in the intravaginal pH to > 4 Gardnerella vaginalis is the most frequently detected BV-causing bacterium. Treatment is with antibiotics such as metronidazole, clindamycin or tinidazole, used orally or vaginally.
- **Yeast Infection**
  - This involves a fungus called Candida albican, or any of several species of candida. You always have some candida in your vagina, but an overgrowth causes yeast infections and symptoms of vaginitis. Treatment is with antifungal clotrimazole or fenticonazole pessaries, creams used vaginally or oral antifungal medication such as fluconazole or itraconazole.

- **Trichomoniasis**
  - This is a type of vaginitis that comes from a tiny, one-celled parasite called Trichomonas vaginalis. Treatment is with oral metronidazole or tinidazole.

Symptoms such as an abnormal discharge, fishy odour, internal or external itching or a vulvovaginal rash suggest a need for medical treatment. With yeast infections and trichomoniasis, it is important to simultaneously treat your partner if you are sexually active and not using barrier protection.

Probiotics have a positive effect on the vaginal microflora by promoting the proliferation of beneficial bacteria such as lactobacilli and altering the intravaginal microbiota composition. There are specialized probiotics for vaginal protection, and they reduce the symptoms of infections and are helpful for the treatment and prevention of BV and VVC.

8

Sexuality, Sexual Health and Well-Being

'We do not have to spend money and go hungry and struggle and study to become sensual. We always were. We need not believe we must somehow earn good erotic care. We always deserved it.'

—Naomi Wolf

I got divorced and, yes, did date. However, I always knew I could bring myself pleasure anytime I wanted. Dr Nozer and I never discussed this subject until a friend of mine, who is also single, visited him and then narrated this story to me much later. She said she was grumbling to Dr Nozer about how she had had to hang up her sex life and has been so devoid of sex that she thought her vagina needed to be dusted, *to which Dr Nozer said, 'well why don't you get a vibrator?'*

First, I fell off the chair laughing and second, I could not believe that Dr Nozer would himself suggest this option. Well, that's just the kind of doctor he is. But for me there was another takeaway. Your doctor should be your champion—sensitive and understanding of your situation and relating to you totally, one-on-one. You should feel secure in having any discussion about you as a woman and your sexual and reproductive health and leave with better understanding or a solution.

Shonali Sabherwal

D was forty-one years old when she first met me, fourteen years ago. She was a single mother, a year into menopause and a fitness buff, committed to aerobic exercise and weight training. She looked and dressed like a woman much younger than her age. She was petrified of ageing prematurely and I started her on hormone therapy via an estrogen patch and oral progesterone with a five-year horizon. Due to the withdrawal of the estrogen patch from the local market a few years into treatment, she was shifted to conventional estrogen-progesterone therapy and she exercised the choice of continuing MHT for a longer term with regular follow up. During this time, she

> *was in a relationship with a younger partner, with concerns about painful sex and diminished libido. After ten years of MHT, she was shifted to tibolone, with local use of visnadine gel to improve libido and pleasure. She was advised lubricants to make sex comfortable and diligent condom use to protect her from infections. After all these years, D weighs almost the same and continues to look younger than her age. She has an active sex life and is for me a role model who projects self-preservation, physical fitness and confidence in addressing her sexuality.*
>
> *Nozer Sheriar*

Sexuality in Midlife

It is a common misconception that menopause causes a decline in sexual desire, response, behaviour and satisfaction. In reality, the female body remains capable of responding to sexual stimuli, albeit with some changes that are important to understand and address. Most women can continue to experience sexual pleasure as they age. In fact, some women report an increase in sexual enjoyment.

Human sexuality is influenced by a multiplicity of factors: physical, hormonal, emotional, as also relationships and personal comfort, confidence or inhibition. These influences continue during the perimenopause, with some of the physical and emotional changes impacting many of these factors positively or negatively.

Know Thyself

Parts of your body with high concentrations of nerve endings can provide pleasurable sensations that are a part of sexual response when stimulated. These are called erogenous zones and they play an important role all through your life. Awareness, consciousness and application of these by you and your partner is always important.

- **Nonspecific erogenous zones** include the skin on the sides and back of the neck, the inner arms, the fingertips, the chest, the abdomen and the thighs. Stimulation of these can heighten sensual response and plays an important role in foreplay.

Figure 11: Knowing the external genitalia

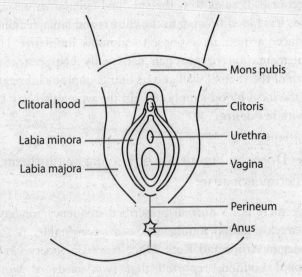

Mons pubis

Clitoral hood

Clitoris

Labia minora

Urethra

Labia majora

Vagina

Perineum

Anus

- **Specific erogenous zones** are directly associated with sexual response and include the lips and nipples in addition to the genitals. On the genitals, the clitoris, the rest of vulva, lower third of the vagina (close to the entrance) and the perineal skin behind the vagina have a higher density of nerves and blood supply. These, when stimulated, can provide pleasurable sensations and lead to sexual arousal and enjoyment.

Why Do Sexual Responses Change?

The changes in response to arousal and sex may be attributed to the many physical and hormonal changes in perimenopause. The deficiency of estrogen causes vaginal dryness, thinning of the vaginal wall and a lack of lubrication, which may result in physical discomfort during intercourse. Besides this, the subdued circulatory response causes less blood flowing to the clitoris and labia, leading to a reduced arousal in response to stimulus and desire. Here, supplementation of estrogen can really help restore the health of the vaginal wall and its lining, improve lubrication and the local blood supply to help the woman's body keep up with her desire.

How Does the Frequency of Having Sex Influence the Perimenopause?

While there is no normal prescribed frequency for having sex, weekly sexual indulgence seems reasonable. A study by Megan Arnot and Ruth Mace from University College Hospital London, reported that two thirds of women engaged in some sort of sexual activity, which included oral sex, caressing and masturbation, on a weekly basis. They found that women who engaged in weekly sexual activity were less likely to experience early menopause and menopause related complaints than those who had sex less than once a month.

Many women in and after the perimenopause remain sexually active, with half in their fifties and a third in their seventies continuing to have sex one way or another. Of course, there are changes and you don't have to expect the same type of sex you were having when you were younger. While there is no worry about your periods, becoming pregnant or being walked in on by your kids, perimenopause is also the stage of life with redefined roles, lowered desire, harder arousal and vaginal dryness which may cause painful intercourse. What earlier felt good may change when getting aroused or having an orgasm becomes difficult. At this time, more mental engagement, gentleness and sensitivity and physical stimulation focused on the clitoris, breasts and other parts of the body could help. Communication remains the key in setting realistic expectations and for couples who either don't have sex or have sex only occasionally, sexual intimacy may simply be cuddling, sharing a bed and laughing together. Every woman has to have the self-confidence to take control and make decisions about her sexuality, type of sex, its frequency and what works best for her.

How Do You Deal with Diminished Drive and Libido?

Libido is essentially a brain function responsive to the sex hormones. While low doses of estrogen prime the brain cells, progesterone is what helps turn the sex drive on. Besides the dance between estrogen and progesterone, testosterone plays a particularly important role in a woman's libido. This is why in some women, the relative shift of balance to testosterone due to a drop in estrogen levels after menopause, actually increases sexual desire and pleasure. Hormones secreted by the adrenal glands contribute to the sex drive and these are affected by emotional and physical stresses. This is why recognizing and addressing psychological problems and lifestyle issues can play an important role in addressing concerns about libido.

Usually, when ovarian function is compromised with adrenal glands being pushed, testosterone levels start dwindling. In post-menopausal women, the ovary has been known to secrete some testosterone and in situations where testosterone levels are low, supplementation has been shown to positively impact libido and improve sexual drive.

How Are Relationships Connected to Sexual Health?

Although sexual behaviour and desires change with age, the need for intimacy and physical closeness does not dissipate. Women can use perimenopause as a time to redefine relationships, particularly sexual relationships. A sex drive that is waning may be the first sign that your relationship is also going through a rough time.

What we are increasingly seeing is that the world of constant stimuli with easy access to gadgets, phones, tablets and social media, keeps people busy and takes over their lives, keeping them away from their relationships. Besides this, in their earlier years, women are primary caregivers, and always putting themselves last.

There is such a thing as 'caregiver burnout'. When a woman finally says, 'I have had enough,' her partner and family may not always respond with the support she deserves. She is fully stressed out by the time she reaches the perimenopause, her adrenal glands being pushed and her cortisol levels either too low or too high. Sexual activity at this time is a function of how healthy you are, how much in balance your hormones are, the relationship you have with your partner and your perception of menopause and libido. Christiane Northrup says:

Sexual function is a complex, integrated phenomenon that reflects the health and balance not only of the ovaries and hormones but also of the cardiovascular system, the brain, the spinal cord, and the peripheral nerves. In addition, every factor that affects sexual function has underlying psychological, sociocultural, interpersonal, and biological influences of its own. Happily, current research on women and sex is finally taking into account how complex female sexual arousal really is. Consequently, the entire concept of so-called female sexual dysfunction is being updated. New research (much of it done by women) is shedding increasing light on how seamlessly psychological states affect biological responses. Finally research has begun to validate what women already know: a woman's experience of sexual arousal is more influenced by her thoughts and emotions than by feedback from her genitals. In other words, her emotions and thoughts must be in sync with the goal of sexual satisfaction for her body to perform sexually. [*]

She further states that this change in sex drive often has absolutely nothing to do with hormone levels and everything to do with a woman's deepest unfulfilled desires, desires that

---

[*] Northrup, Christiane, *The Wisdom of Menopause*, Hay House, 2012, p. 322.

are now rising into her consciousness. She mentions that women have two hearts. The heart in the chest is the high heart and the uterus and genitals are the low heart. The high heart and the low heart are energetically connected. During midlife, the dictates of your high heart's desires become increasingly urgent, and your low heart and genitals will no longer willingly participate in sex that is not connected to your high heart and your deepest yearnings. Which means, many women need love and intimacy than just routine sex.

How Do You Recognize Female Sexual Dysfunction?

Sexual dysfunction in women typically presents as loss of desire, decreased arousal, inability to reach orgasm and sexual pain; and these frequently overlap. While sexual dysfunction can occur at any age, women in the menopausal transition and beyond tend to experience sexual, health-related conditions or concerns more often. While female sexual dysfunction is distressing for many women and warrants medical attention, sexual dysfunction in general, is often minimized due to cultural stigma. Treatment of sexual dysfunction can be complex and often requires a multidisciplinary approach. Doctors should thus have a low threshold for appropriate referral to the proper specialists.

There are four common categories of female sexual dysfunction:

- **Low Sexual Desire**
  - Loss of sexual desire in women can be distressing and is the most common of the sexual disorders in women. Causes include medical conditions, hormonal change, medications such as antidepressants,

antipsychotics or opioids and psychosocial factors like untreated anxiety and depression or a history of sexual abuse.

- **Low Arousal**
  o Low arousal, difficulty or inability to become or stay physically aroused or excited during sexual activity can present as a decrease in vaginal lubrication or genital warmth due to decreased blood flow. Low arousal states can be due to hypertension, hyperlipidaemia or diabetes and should be treated. Low arousal may be related to hormonal changes following menopause. A decrease in estrogen leads to decreased blood flow to the pelvic region, which can result in less genital sensation, as well as needing more time to build arousal and reach orgasm.

- **Orgasmic Dysfunction**
  o Some women complain of delayed, less intense or absent orgasm, which can be lifelong or acquired. In women, orgasmic dysfunction often occurs with sexual pain or poor arousal. The doctor should identify any psychosocial contributors.

- **Sexual Pain**
  o Sexual pain refers to the pain associated with sexual stimulation or vaginal contact. Sexual pain is common among women of all ages and includes vulvar pain (vulvodynia), deep pain with penetration (dyspareunia) or tightening of the pelvic musculature (vaginismus). Many conditions can cause sexual pain, including insufficient lubrication, vulvar skin lesions such as lichen sclerosis and lichen planus, pelvic floor muscle abnormalities leading to deeper

pelvic pain and endocrine abnormalities such as low testosterone.

Whither Self-Pleasure? To Do or Not to Do?

Most women feel ashamed and embarrassed at bringing up the subject of self-pleasure with masturbation. Although all men and most women pleasure themselves, we still don't want to admit to it. So here again it's better to bring in a real story—mine.

I've always felt that I may be having too much libido. I discovered, when I was thirteen, that I could bring myself to achieve an orgasm, no one told me how. My mother and father never dealt with this subject, and it just unfolded the way any kid's sexuality unfolds over time. As I experienced love at a young age, the natural progression of a loving relationship made me experience sex in a different light.

We started this chapter with the interaction with my friend, so when we were writing this book, I asked Dr Nozer 'Do you think we should cover masturbation?'

And he said, 'Yes, of course, we cannot leave it out.'

Shonali Sabherwal

Masturbation is normal and natural and does not require any reasoning or justification, let alone any guilt. Women, like men, indulge in masturbation and experiment with it at different times in their sexual journey. Yet, they have been conditioned to keep doubting themselves and questioning their normalcy.

Even so, there are many, evidence-based benefits of self-pleasure, which also come into play during perimenopause:

- Busts stress and releases tension.
- Elevates mood and boosts concentration.
- Benefits sleep.
- Allows women to understand and know what to expect from partners.
- Keeps the pelvic floor strong.
- It is supposed to boost immune function.
- It promotes a balance of neurotransmitters, dopamine, oxytocin and decreases cortisol.

Snapshot on Lifestyle and Diet

Lifestyle Recommendations

- Communicate with your partner about what you want and what he or she wants. It's important to share.
- Make more time for lovemaking. In today's world, this is a huge problem.
- Focus on foreplay. Women want this (don't you agree?) and if men don't know, make them read this—foreplay is like prepping a woman and they'll thank you for it!
- Try massage, erotica and new-for-you sex routines as ways to build desire.
- Include Kegel exercises (see exercise section). These are by far the best to keep you all toned from the inside.
- Exercise to release endorphins (feel-good hormones). I cannot stress enough the importance of exercise, not

just to look great but to enhance muscle tone and your performance.

- Try couple therapy if things get really tough in the bedroom.
- Manage and reduce stress, as this is a big deterrent when it comes to having sex.

Diet Recommendations

How you are in the bedroom, and your moods that affect libido definitely get influenced by the foods you eat, as foods have their own energy. All the dietary recommendations below stem from eliminating or minimizing foods that would cause your libido to plummet and and decrease the inflammation underlying almost all conditions, underlying almost all conditions. Macrobiotic philosophy focuses on eating too many foods of one nature, which causes you to compensate by craving foods of the opposite nature. I have also explained this in the diet section of the book.

- Quit sugar and this includes refined white flour (maida) or products off the shelf that have hidden sugars. Sugar plays havoc with the system. It not only causes an acidic blood condition and robs you of gut bacteria, but also makes you go through sugar highs and lows, so when you hit a low the energy just drops. This will cause you to be lethargic, unresponsive and unready for action.
- Decrease caffeinated drinks. These will give you an artificial high and then cause your energy to drop.
- Quit processed foods, as hidden sugars will also cause imbalances in sexual energy.

- Quit smoking as it dehydrates you, upsetting the body's basal temperature and the body does not have adequate circulation.
- Minimize eating too much dairy, as dairy does not get totally absorbed by the body and the residue tends to cause the blood to get acidic, interfering with the flow of blood to the genitals and extremities.
- Minimize animal protein (meats) as it tends to digest slowly and cause an acidic blood condition impacting energy levels.
- Minimize having too much fruit juices. Fruit is fine but having fruit juices where more than one fruit is used to make a juice is too much fructose for the body to handle which the body then treats as it would sugar, depleting sexual energy.
- Increase the consumption of complex carbohydrates like brown rice and millets as this will not only aid the digestive system, but also keep your sugars steady, bringing in the energy you need for activity, including sex.
- Stick to a balanced diet of grains, vegetables, beans, nuts, seeds, fruits, fermented foods and stay mostly plant-based.
- Use turmeric as it is an inflammatory and will help control all the other negatives that come in when eating goes haywire. Use it in moderation. The way we Indians use it as a part of our Indian cooking is adequate.

A Few Love-Foods and Antioxidants That Can Help Boost Sexual Energy

- Lycopene, the pinkish-red carotenoid in tomatoes, papaya, watermelons and grapefruit.

- Lutein and zeaxanthin, found in dark green vegetables, broccoli, green and yellow peppers, corn, kinnow and goji berries (native to Tibet, China and also India).
- Proanthocyanidins, found in green vegetables, red wine and grape juice.
- Resveratrol, found in red wine, red grapes, green tea, and cacao powder.
- Flavonoids, found in red wine, citrus fruits and dark chocolate.
- Lignans, found in flax seeds, sesame seeds, some whole grains (barley, wheat and whole oats), cruciferous vegetables like cauliflower and broccoli; apricots, strawberries and soybean.
- Vitamin C, found in tomatoes, citrus fruits, peppers, potatoes, broccoli, gooseberry (amla), lychee and green chillies.
- Indole carbinol 3, found in cruciferous vegetables like cauliflower, cabbage and broccoli.
- Carotenoids, of which beta carotene is the major one, found in pumpkin, sweet potatoes and yellow vegetables like yellow peppers or cantaloupe.
- $(1\rightarrow3)$-β-D-Glucan, found in whole oats (not rolled oats), barley and maitake mushrooms. More concentrated in the outer layers of any cereal grain, also referred to as bran.
- Ellagic acid, found in strawberries, walnuts, apples, pomegranate, raspberries and grapes.
- Vitamin E, found in wheat germ, sunflower and safflower oils, avocados, asparagus, sweet potato, broccoli, nuts (of which almonds have the highest amount), the tops of turnips (shalgam), tomatoes, pine nuts (chilgoza a rich source of minerals, protein, zinc

and magnesium) and shrimp (an excellent source of zinc and magnesium).

- Selenium is a trace mineral from nuts, liver, sunflower seeds, fish, all grain brans, spirulina, shitake mushroom, onions, goji berries, celery, sesame seeds and fish. It is required in small quantities and is required for endurance.

- Superoxide dismutase (SOD), catalase (CAT) and glutathione peroxidase, and oxidized lipids (fats). SOD foods include wheat grass, barley grass, broccoli and cabbage and CAT foods include wheat sprouts, potatoes and carrots.

- Alpha-Lipoic Acid (ALA) protects your cells as all antioxidants do. It is responsible for energy exchange between cells and works as a support to glutathione, vitamins C and E when these wear themselves out by fighting the free radicals. ALA is found in lysine (an amino acid) and is bound to protein, essentially in meats, broccoli, spinach and brewer's yeast.

- Co Q-10 found in wheat germ (or other germ portions of grains), fish seeds, nuts, canola and soybean oils, broccoli, cauliflower, strawberries (which also have iron, beta-carotene, folic acid, vitamin E, calcium, and magnesium) and oranges. Required for the small mitochondria in cells where we produce energy.

- Anthocyanins are red to blue pigments found in foods, more concentrated in black-coloured foods. Anthocyanins are found in berries like blueberries, cranberries, black and red raspberries, cherries, red cabbage, black soybean and black grapes.

- Fish is an excellent low-fat source of powerful protein and Omega 3 and great polyunsaturated oils (PUFAs).

Fish oils help in endothelial functioning and enhance nitric oxide (NO). While we do not advocate going off animal foods completely for non-vegetarians, we do advocate achieving a balance with animal foods, chicken, eggs and dairy; moderation is the name of the game.

- Coconut oil is known to increase energy as it does not require bile for digestion, and the body turns fatty acids into energy right away.

- Saffron (kesar) is known to be sexually stimulating; it improves blood circulation and helps the kidneys.

- Nutmeg (jaiphal) is known to stimulate nerve cells and aid blood circulation.

- Basil stimulates sex drive and boosts fertility.

- Maca, a Peruvian plant, can be used in powder form. An aphrodisiac among the Incas, it has a chemical called p-methoxybenzyl isothiocyanate, which is known to enhance sexual drive.

- Chocolate is also referred to as nutritional gold. It is a powerful antioxidant and is known to stimulate endorphins, putting you in a positive state of mind by enhancing serotonin.

- Siberian ginseng and shilajit are aphrodisiacs.

- Chromium boosts metabolism by enhancing the action of insulin and zinc.

Medical Management to Support and Maintain Sexual Health

General Quality of Sex Life in the Menopause

Sexual wellbeing remains relevant to the general quality of life as one ages; sexuality is still important to many elderly women before menopause and beyond. As we have already read, age and declining levels of sex hormones have detrimental effects on sexual functioning, with a significant increase in vaginal dryness and painful sex (dyspareunia) and a significant decrease in desire and sexual responsiveness.

Psychological and relational factors are very important, influencing sexual symptoms and the level of distress in post-menopausal women.

- A woman's sexual response to her partner is significantly related to her baseline feelings for the partner, their relationship qualities and the partner's age and health.
- A good doctor will include appropriate questions to investigate sexual wellbeing because women may not be willing to initiate a conversation on sexual interest, behaviour and activity themselves, but they usually appreciate being questioned by doctors.
- It is equally important for a woman to raise and discuss issues related to her sexual health with her doctor and to expect sensitivity, support, guidance and medical assistance.

No one should believe that sex is not important for elderly women and both women and their doctors should make the effort and take the initiative to break the ice and have a dialogue on sexual health.

Hormone Therapy

The pivotal role of GSM should be always considered because the two most common symptoms, vaginal dryness and dyspareunia, may affect other sexual responses, the desire, arousal and orgasm satisfaction, as well as cause pelvic floor dysfunction.

MHT with estrogens alone or in combination with progestogens when used in women with menopausal symptoms, will be associated with a small to moderate improvement in sexual function, particularly in the pain aspect. Tibolone, a form of MHT is a selective tissue estrogenic activity regulator (STEAR), is of value in treating post-menopausal women with female sexual dysfunction (FSD).

Women's sexuality is multidimensional and hormonal and non-hormonal treatments and psychosexual strategies should be individualized and tailored according to a woman's history and current needs, taking into account also the partner's availability, general and sexual health of the partner and quality of the intimate relationship.

Androgen Therapy in the Perimenopause

Androgen levels decline with age in women with the greatest decline observed during perimenopause. There is strong evidence that androgens influence female sexual function, and that testosterone therapy may be useful for women who have experienced loss of sexual desire and/or arousal.

The primary indication for using testosterone is for the treatment of diminished sexual desire that is causing the affected woman to experience significant distress. Before testosterone therapy is considered, other causes of impaired sexual desire and/or arousal, such as dyspareunia, depression, medication side-effects, relationship issues and other health problems affecting the woman or her partner, should be addressed.

Most recently, hypoactive sexual desire disorder (HSDD) and sexual arousal disorder have been re-classified as a single entity, sexual interest-arousal disorder, since it is recognized that arousal and desire are closely interlinked. Testosterone therapy improves both desire and arousal. Testosterone gel may be used transdermal or intravaginally, alone or with vaginal estrogen. It has been shown to improve painful sex, sexual desire, lubrication and satisfaction. Beneficial effects have been seen with administration thrice a week.

Side-effects of testosterone therapy are dose-related and avoidable with the use of formulations and doses appropriate for women. Testosterone therapy may be started as a clinical trial after counselling and may be discontinued if a woman has not experienced significant benefit within six months.

Newer Treatments for Sexual Health in Women

As per research by Cleveland Clinic, Ohio, about 43 per cent of women and 31 per cent of men say they experience some degree of sexual dysfunction and along with it, stigma.

1. In 2013, the FDA approved ospemifene (Osphena) for moderate to severe painful intercourse in women.
2. In 2015, the FDA green-lighted flibanserin (Addyi) for low sexual desire in pre-menopausal women.
3. In 2019 the FDA approved bremelanotide (Vyleesi) for pre-menopausal women with low sexual desire.

We await most of these medications for use in clinical practice in India.

Management of Female Sexual Dysfunction

Low Sexual Desire

Treatment often entails a multidisciplinary approach:

- Sex education and counselling.
- Sildenafil in a low dose has been used but with mixed results.
- Medications like the above-mentioned FDA-approved flibanserin and bremelanotide for pre-menopausal women.
- Hormone therapy such as estrogen, testosterone or ospemifene if sexual pain is related to low desire.
- A vaginal insert called prasterone (Intrarosa), a DHEA supplement.
- Lifestyle remedies like stress reduction and planning and taking time for sexual intimacy.

Sexual Pain

Treatment depends on the cause:

- Vulvar physiotherapy.
- Partnered dilator therapy.
- Hyaluronic acid gel to moisturize the vulvovaginal epithelium.
- Lubrication is a fast and easy way to get your wetness back. It relieves vaginal dryness that can lead to friction, burning and pain during intercourse. There are a lot of lubes on the market. You may need to try a few to find one that works for you. You need to put it in your vagina and on your partner's penis, fingers, or a toy each time you have sex.

- o Water-based lubes (KY jelly, Lubic jelly) work well if you need to lessen a lot of friction. But you may have to reapply during sex.
- o Silicone-based lubes (Astroglide, Penchant gel) last longer than lubes made from water. They also more expensive. Since silicone can stain your sheets, you may want to put a towel down.
- Local anaesthetic gels.
- Superficial ulceration of the lower margin of vaginal opening (fourchette) happens due to friction during sex due to vaginal atrophy.
  - o Water-based vaginal lubricants to reduce vaginal dryness and discomfort.
  - o Treat with local antibiotic cream for healing the abrasion.
  - o May be avoided by varying the position during penetration to avoid pressure on the fourchette (the posterior margin of the vagina).
  - o Placing a pillow under the hips will also help protect the fourchette by changing the alignment.
- Ospemifene for moderate to severe painful intercourse.
- Prasterone (Intrarosa) vaginal capsules to relieve dyspareunia.
- Local hormone treatment with intravaginal testosterone and estradiol-releasing vaginal rings.
- Vaginal laser therapy is also being researched to make the vaginal lining healthier.

Low Arousal

Referral to specialists in sexual health.

- Cognitive behavioural therapy may also be helpful.

- In some women with low arousal sildenafil has shown some efficacy.

Orgasmic Dysfunction

Treatment for orgasmic dysfunction is challenging. Some things that can help:

- Mindfulness training.
- Yoga.
- Directed masturbation.
- Use of sex toys and sex therapy.
- If you are comfortable with the idea, you can explore the use of vibrators, dildos or masturbation sleeves to give you more options for pleasure.
- Because selective serotonin reuptake inhibitors (SSRIs) can affect orgasms their doses can be reduced.
- Testosterone supplementation, dopamine agonists and sildenafil have been used.

Management of Male Sexual Dysfunction

Sexuality cannot be seen in isolation and the effect of sexual dysfunction in the male partner can be an important contributing factor. In 1998, the FDA approved sildenafil (Viagra) for erectile dysfunction and since then, thanks to a marketing blitz from pharmaceutical companies and new medicines, the topic of male sexual dysfunction has moved into the mainstream.

While men do not have a clear hormonal demarcation in their midlife there is no doubt that low testosterone levels do impact their reproductive and sexual health in what is sometimes referred to as the 'andropause'. This is also the time where physical health issues such as diabetes and hypertension, medications for hypertension or depression, smoking, alcoholism and substance abuse can result in erectile dysfunction. Psychological issues may arise from performance anxiety, marital and relationship problems and stress in personal and professional lives.

The main types of male sexual dysfunction in midlife are:

- Erectile dysfunction—difficulty in getting or keeping an erection.
- Low libido—a reduced interest in sex.

Most cases of male sexual dysfunction can be corrected by treating the mental or physical problems that cause it:

- Drugs exist to help improve sexual function by increasing blood flow to the penis. Sildenafil (Viagra) and tadalafil (Cialis) are safe and effective for most men and have transformed the treatment of erectile dysfunction.
- Low levels of testosterone are treated by hormone-replacement therapies using oral medication, gels or injections and have a positive effect on libido.
- Counselling may help address feelings of anxiety, depression, fear or guilt that may affect sexual function.

Sexual dysfunction in midlife is a couple issue and often has both a female and a male component. Treatment has to be thoughtful and supportive and holistic, often needing more than just medication. It needs communication, sensitivity, mutual respect and caring between partners.

9

Bone Health

'These fragments I have shored against my ruins.'

—T.S. Eliot

A while ago, my friend, Puja, was staying over at my place, and we were lying down and chatting in my bed. Suddenly I sat up but took two minutes to stand up, and then when I walked to the loo, I walked like my grandmother. She started laughing and said to me, 'you look like my nani.' Now this is me, someone who exercises like a horse, eats well and does a lot of meditation. Over time I have worked hard at keeping my bones healthy. I should have strong bones, right?

The grandmother walk was possibly a hard workout on that day, and this usually happens if one engages in an intense yoga routine or workout. But

I also do realize the fragility of my own bones as I approach menopause.

The moral of the story? Keep working out and stay away from sugar.

Shonali Sabherwal

A was forty-one years old when she first came to consult me, seven years ago. She presented with irregular menses and excessive facial hair with a diagnosis of both hypothyroidism and polycystic ovarian syndrome (PCOS). She had previously been treated with oral contraceptive pills containing cyproterone and an antiandrogen flutamide. Her FSH levels off the pill were 2.3 and estradiol, 192, and with menopause being sometime away she was advised a low-dose oral contraceptive pill with drosperinone for birth control, regular periods and cosmetic benefit. A baseline bone density (DEXA) at this time reported low bone mass of -1.7 (osteopenia) in her lower spine for which she was advised weight bearing exercise, calcium and vitamin D supplements and periodic vigilance. She took a break from the contraceptive pill four years later and started experiencing excessive perspiration, hair loss and bone pain. At this time, her FSH levels at 21 suggested she was in perimenopause, for which she was advised to resume the birth-control pills which she could take up to the age of fifty. A repeat DEXA reported a reduction in density to -2.4 for which she *was now prescribed 150 mg risedronate once a month, from a class of medications called bisphosphonates. She has continued on these medications to date and is symptom free. A recent DEXA scan showed no further bone loss, but in fact an improvement of bone density to -2. There being issues with long term bisphosphonate use, the medication has to be assessed periodically and will be stopped at five years of use. Bone health is probably one of the most important components of perimenopause care, yet neglected and overlooked.*

Nozer Sheriar

Your Skeletal System

The bones in your body are a living tissue that grow and renew themselves throughout your life. Bones allow you to support yourself and your weight. They are designed for compressive strength, the application of weight, force and tensile strength. This strength is contributed by their calcium carbonate and phosphate content.

There are two types of bone cells that you should know of: osteoclasts and osteoblasts. Osteoclasts do all the repair work in your body, travelling through your body looking for older bone in need of revival, dissolving and absorbing it and leaving spaces behind. These are then filled by the osteoblasts, which produce new bone to fill these spaces, a process called remodelling. If these two functions stay in balance, we have good bone mass and bone strength. Osteoporosis is a result of osteoclast dominance, where more bone is being dissolved and reabsorbed and less bone is being generated.

Bone metabolism thus is a complex process in which construction and demolition crews work side by side. When you are young, the bone builders outnumber the bone destroyers. But the balance shifts as you get older. A wide variety of conditions, including deficiency of vitamin D and bone-building minerals, a high-acid diet and steroid use, can allow the osteoclasts, the cells that break down bone to outpace the osteoblasts, the cells that make bone. The result is weakened bones.

Your bones are also homes for essential minerals, especially calcium, which is responsible for a lot of functions in your body, including helping muscles contract, regulating heartbeat, aiding clotting of blood, keeping your joints free of inflammation and helping your brain communicate with your nerves by releasing neurotransmitters. The amount of calcium required to do these functions is 1 per cent of your stores. The rest of the 1–2 kg worth of calcium is stored in your bone and when the supply of calcium in your blood drops, it is taken from the stores in your bone.

Over her lifetime, a woman may lose almost 40 per cent of peak bone mass while a man may lose just 20 per cent of his. So, although men and women both lose bone, the menopausal acceleration of bone loss, as illustrated in the chart, suggests that the decline in sex hormones is the cause of this differential between women and men.

What Is Osteopenia and Osteoporosis?

Probably the most significant medical conditions and health hazards that women experience during perimenopause are

Figure 12: Differential bone loss between women and men

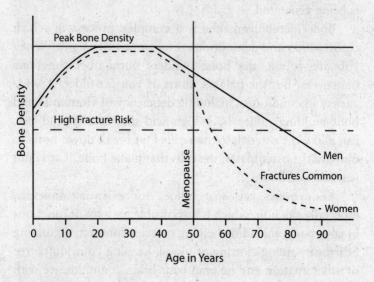

osteopenia and osteoporosis. While both women and men lose bone mass as they age, women lose mass by 0.5 to 3 per cent each year immediately after menopause, resulting in an over 40 per cent loss during the rest of their lives. The fractures that result from weakened bone are, for the older woman, the most important threat to her health and her life. Osteoporosis is a common metabolic disease in India, and it is estimated that 46 million women over the age of fifty live with it. The prevalence of low bone mass in Indian women is to the extent of 40 per cent at the age of forty, 62 per cent by the age of sixty and 80 per cent by the age of sixty-five.

Osteoporosis is a systemic skeletal disease characterized by diminished bone strength with the risk of sustaining a fracture when falling from own body height (fragility fracture). Osteopenia is when your bones are weaker than normal but not so far gone that they break easily, which is the hallmark of osteoporosis. It as a midpoint between healthy bones and osteoporosis. Bone strength is determined by a combination of bone density and bone structure (microarchitectural integrity). Post-menopausal osteoporosis results from a failure to attain peak bone density, accelerated bone loss after menopause, age-related bone loss or a combination of factors. Accelerated, post-menopausal bone loss is induced by a fall in estrogen levels.

Figure 13: Differences between normal and osteoporotic bone

Electron micrography of trabecular bone

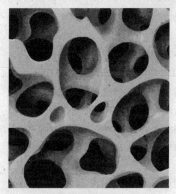   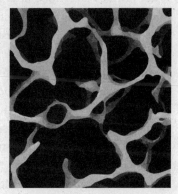

Normal bone   Osteoporotic bone

Decreased bone mass is also the result of your diet, deficiencies of calcium, vitamin D and magnesium, levels of estrogen, testosterone, thyroid hormone and insulin, and hormones like norepinephrine and cortisol (stress hormone).

Estrogen has a beneficial role in osteoporosis; MHT advised and monitored by a doctor is definitely associated with fewer fractures. Although skeletal health is a function of your genetic predisposition, it can be modified by lifestyle factors such as diet, weight-bearing exercise, avoidance of bone-toxic substances and a healthy approach to menopause.

How Do You Diagnose Osteopenia and Osteoporosis?

The diagnosis of osteoporosis is based on assessment of bone mineral density (BMD) by an imaging technique called dual X-ray absorptiometry (DXA) or dual energy X-ray absorptiometry (DEXA). The value obtained is compared to peak bone density and expressed as the T-score. Osteoporosis is defined at a T-score of -2.5 or the presence of a fragility fracture. Assessment of BMD may be used for routine screening, but is best applied on a selective basis, based on age and other risk factors such as a personal or family history of fractures, history of amenorrhea, primary ovarian insufficiency, low body mass, diet, smoking, alcohol abuse, the use of bone-toxic medication and rheumatoid arthritis. An appropriate assessment of prevalent fractures and secondary causes of osteoporosis should precede any treatment.

Monitoring of treatment by serial DXA is useful, but should be interpreted with caution, taking into account the site monitored, the time interval between scans and drug-specific expectations. Repeat DXA scan should be performed at the same centre to improve accuracy and efficacy.

- If T score > -1, without risk factors, repeat after five years.
- If T score < -1 but > -2.5. with risk factors but not on treatment, repeat every two years.

- If T score < -2.5, with progressive disease on treatment, repeat every year until stable and earlier if clinical situation warrants.

What are fragility fractures?

These are fractures that result from mechanical forces or injuries that would not ordinarily result in a fracture (such as a fall from a standing height or less). Reduced bone density is a major risk factor for fragility fractures, which occur most commonly in the spine, hip and wrist. Hip fracture is responsible for the largest proportion of fractures, even more so in elderly women. By predisposing to hip, vertebral and other related fractures, osteoporosis places tremendous health and financial burden on individuals and on healthcare systems.

How Do You Determine Your Risk for Osteoporosis?

Listed here are the predisposing factors that have been identified to increase the risk of osteopenia and osteoporosis. Contained in these risks are also strategies to protect yourself.

- A family history, particularly if your mother has been diagnosed with osteoporosis or has had a hip or an osteoporotic fracture.
- You are lean with less than 18 per cent body fat, since you need body fat to manufacture estrogen in the perimenopause.
- You smoke, since smoking hastens menopause by one to two years, as it decreases hormone levels prematurely.

Estrogen, testosterone and progesterone all protect bone.

- You spend most of your time indoors since women who are not exposed to natural sunlight are deficient in the vitamin D necessary for bone mineralization.

- You are sedentary and spend fewer than four hours per day on your feet. A sedentary lifestyle provides insufficient weight-bearing exercise to stimulate bone growth. Weight training has shown to build bone density even in perimenopausal women who are not on estrogen.

- You are, or were, a fitness fanatic, with a lifestyle that includes dieting for weight loss and engaging regularly in strenuous exercise such as marathon training. Dietary restrictions and the chronic stress of overtraining can impair mineral absorption. It also disrupts the hypothalamic-pituitary-ovarian (HPO) axis, which is the exquisite feedback loop between the brain, the body and our hormone levels. Chronic over-exercise without adequate caloric or mineral intake results in stress fractures in ballet dancers, gymnasts, soccer players and competitive runners, among others.

- You have a history of no periods associated with excessive exercise or the eating disorder anorexia nervosa. This too is associated with a derangement of the HPO axis, resulting in lower estrogen, androgen and progesterone, inhibiting your body's ability to lay down new bone and to remodel old bone.

- You drink more than 2.5 g of alcohol per day. Alcohol interferes with the function of both osteoblasts and osteoclasts, inhibiting your ability to lay down new bone and to remodel old bone. There are 10 g servings of alcohol in:

o Beer—350 ml
o Wine—120 ml
o Beverage 80 proof—50 ml

- Your liver is overstressed. Its ability to produce and metabolize estrogen is essential for the growth and maintenance of strong bones at any age. Drinking more than two alcoholic drinks per day, taking medication known to be hard on the liver such as statins to lower cholesterols and viral hepatitis are among the significant liver stressors.

- You drink more than two units of caffeine per day. Caffeine results in increased urinary excretion of calcium so the more you consume, the more calcium you lose. However, if your calcium and mineral intake are high, a couple of cups of coffee a day are fine.

  o 250 ml coffee is 1 unit of caffeine.
  o 350 ml tea is 0.4 units of caffeine.
  o Even though tea contains caffeine, both green and black tea have been shown to build bone mass because of their phytoestrogen content.

- You have been clinically depressed for a significant period of time because of the high levels of the immune system chemical known as IL-6, which overstimulates the osteoclasts, cells that break down bone. Depression is also associated with abnormalities in the HPO axis and with elevated cortisol secretion, which predispose one to bone loss.

- Your diet is poor with little fresh food, few leafy green vegetables and lots of fast food. Such a diet does not provide minerals and other nutrients necessary to support the growth and maintenance of a solid bone foundation.

- You went through premature menopause, have had your ovaries removed surgically or went through menopause as a result of radiation or chemotherapy. A woman who enters menopause prematurely for any reason is at an increased risk of osteoporosis unless she gets adequate hormone therapy during the years when her body would normally have produced higher level of hormones.

- You take steroids regularly for conditions such as asthma or lupus. Steroid drugs result in accelerated breakdown of tissue in the body, including the collagen matrix for both skin and bone. They also diminish the sensitivity of the bowel to vitamin D, which in turn reduces calcium absorption. Prolonged use may also significantly decrease estrogen and androgen levels.

- You have taken high doses or been on a long-term regimen of any of the prescription or OTC drugs to block the production of stomach acid, such as used to treat gastroesophageal reflux disease (GERD), stomach and small intestine ulcers and inflammation of the oesophagus. The acid in the stomach is crucial for absorbing bone-building nutrients such as calcium and a deficiency may increase the risk of hip, wrist and spine fractures.

- You have at least two consecutive bone density tests, at least six months apart, done on the same machine that reported scores more than 2.5 standard deviations below normal for your age.

- You have a thyroid disorder, since in hyperthyroidism the excess thyroid hormone stimulates the osteoclasts to break down bone and in hypothyroidism the risk comes from high doses of thyroid medication.

- You are consuming a high-protein diet, the usual recommendation being 40 to 60 grams for adults. Excess protein is excreted through the urine and also increases the urinary excretion of calcium.
- If you are on diuretics (medication to stimulate kidneys to induce micturition), used to treat heart failure, hypertension or fluid retention from any cause.

The use of diuretics correlates with increased fracture risk as they cause an increased urinary excretion of minerals. A better approach to tackle fluid retention would be to follow a diet and avoid salty foods.

- If you have metabolic acidosis, which means an increase of the blood condition being acidic. If this happens, the body uses calcium to bring back the body into balance and this is usually taken from the bones.

How Can We Make Bones Stronger?

One of the myths surrounding osteoporosis is that it is a condition that accompanies menopause. Osteopenia followed by osteoporosis begins long before estrogen levels start to fall and then accelerates for a few years during the perimenopause. Osteoporosis begins anywhere from five to twenty years prior to menopause. So, the better the bones you build when young, the more the benefit you will reap in your later years.

Taking estrogen in the perimenopause can slow down bone loss by a few years, but its effect eventually wears off. Hormone therapy is not the remedy. We are built to maintain strong healthy bones through our adult life and we are also built to withstand normal bone loss as we age. It is our lifestyle—lack of exercise, unhealthy eating habits, lack of sunshine to get vitamin D, fad and yo-yo dieting—that causes loss of bone mass. A healthy lifestyle in your younger years is what will protect your bones as you age.

Snapshot on Lifestyle and Diet

Your bones will respond to the stimuli you give to them, be it through diet, exercise or supplementation. Here are some of the tools that you can adopt and use to build stronger bones.

Lifestyle Recommendations

- Add strength and weight-bearing exercises to your routine, such as weight training, Pilates and/or yoga. Anything that will aid flexibility and involve your bones, muscles, tendons and ligaments is good.

Alignment, posture and flexibility have everything to do with bone mass and strength training, in other words adding some stress on the bones is very important to maintain them.

- Get your vitamin D levels checked periodically. In India, we have an epidemic of vitamin D deficiency, partly due to not getting out in the sun and partly due lack of absorption in the gut of vital nutrients from the foods we eat.
  - o It is beneficial to get out in the sun for twenty to thirty minutes a day without a sunblock on (except on your face), early in the morning or late in the afternoon.

o   Vitamin D is what helps your bones absorb the much-needed calcium, since calcium is not absorbed without sufficient vitamin D in your blood.

- Stop smoking as it gobbles up the calcium and everything else.
- Get your hormone levels checked regularly around the perimenopause. Also, post-menopause, it is good to know where you stand on estrogen and testosterone.

Diet Recommendations

- Make sure you follow a good diet as outlined in this book.
- Minimize alcohol and all other stimulants like caffeine. Alcohol will prevent osteoblast formation, while caffeine is a diuretic that will cause calcium to get excreted through urine.
- Add turmeric to your diet. Shonali eats a raw turmeric (kacha haldi) pickle daily. Of course, it's seasonal, so she buys it in season, or just uses the powder. Add pepper while using turmeric, in the ratio explained in the diet section of this book, to enhance its bioavailability. Its primary active agent, curcumin, has been known to have anti-inflammatory properties.
  o   Curcumin is beneficial in our battle against bad microbes and efforts to create good biodiversity in our gut. It decreases the harmful seepage of toxins from the gut to the human body and helps calm the immune response.
  o   It has been known to help with the generation of more fat storage in the cells and decrease body weight, with a good diet in place.

o   It has been known to elevate tryptophan and serotonin, which help lower appetite.

o   Curcumin increases adiponectin impacting insulin levels. It has been known to have blood thinning qualities, and positively impacts lipid metabolism, helping to lower bad cholesterol.

Supplements

- Include magnesium 400–1000 mg.
- Make sure you supplement the following trace minerals: vitamin C, boron, zinc, manganese, copper, vitamin K2 and calcium.

   o   Vitamin K will boost the effects of vitamin D specially in the lumbar spine. It is found in meat, fermented foods, cheese and other dairy products. If you are a vegan get it from fermented vegetable, kale, seeds, chickpeas and the brassica family of vegetables, broccoli, cauliflower and Brussels sprouts.

   o   High doses of vitamin K can make clotting problems worse, so if you are on blood clotting medicine, please ask your health practitioner before you supplement.

   o   Vitamin K2 is an important form of vitamin K that helps bone health in women at the time of perimenopause and menopause. It is known to slow down the rate of bone weakening at this time, increase bone strength and decrease number of fractures. It boosts the effectiveness of osteoporosis medication.

   o   Add natto (Japanese fermented soybean), a macrobiotic product to boost vitamin K2.

Medical Treatment for Osteopenia and Osteoporosis

Menopause Hormone Therapy

MHT decreases the incidence of all fractures, including vertebral and hip fractures, even in women not at high risk of fracture. It is the only therapy available with proven efficacy of fracture reduction in patients with osteopenia. All types of MHT, including low dose, non-oral routes of estrogen, are effective in preserving bone mass.

- MHT may be used for the prevention and treatment of osteoporosis in the early post-menopause period in symptomatic women unless there is a contraindication.
  - It prevents all osteoporotic fractures even in low-risk population.
  - It increases spine BMD up to 7.5 per cent, femoral neck BMD up to 4.5 per cent over three years and reduces the risk of spine, hip and other osteoporotic fractures by up to 40 per cent.
  - Although MHT prevents fractures at any age after menopause, age at the initiation of MHT is important. In the age group between fifty and sixty years or within ten years after menopause, the benefits of MHT are most likely to outweigh any risk and can be considered as first-line therapy.
  - The fracture protective effect of MHT is limited to standard dosages of estrogen therapy, while that for protection against loss of BMD is available for lower than standard doses.
- Tibolone has an affinity for estrogen, progesterone and androgen receptors and prevents vertebral and non-vertebral fractures.

Calcium and Vitamin D

Post-menopausal women need a daily intake of 1000–1500 mg of elemental calcium. Calcium supplementation should be adjusted to bridge the shortfall between daily requirement and the dietary intake.

The requirement for vitamin D is 800–1000 IU in the post-menopausal period. As the major source of vitamin D is dependent on sunlight exposure, the need for supplementation will vary. Measuring the blood vitamin-D level is helpful in deciding the dose and vitamin-D supplementation has been shown to independently lower the risk of fracture from falling in elderly patients.

Bisphosphonates

Bisphosphonates such as alendronate, residronate and ibandronate are potent inhibitors of bone resorption with proven efficacy in the prevention of vertebral and hip fractures. Due to safety issues and risk of over-suppression of bone turnover following use of bisphosphonates for longer than three to five years, a drug-free period may be considered after three years of intravenous zoledronic acid or five years of oral alendronate therapy.

Bisphosphonates may be associated with flu-like symptoms like headache and myalgia, which are mild and resolve in one to two days. They are taken on an empty stomach and may be associated with severe oesophagitis (inflammation of the oesophagus). Sitting upright, standing or going for a walk for thirty minutes post-medication is a good way to prevent severe acidity and oesophagitis.

Selective Estrogen Receptor Modulators (SERMs)

SERMs, such as raloxifene, reduce vertebral fractures in post-menopausal women with or without prevalent vertebral fractures. SERMs do not alleviate VMS associated with menopause.

Parathyroid Hormone

Parathyroid hormone (PTH) (Forteo) is an anabolic agent that significantly reduces risk of vertebral fractures by stimulation of bone formation. PTH is used in severe osteoporosis or for fracture while on other forms of therapy. PTH is given as a daily subcutaneous injection for a maximum of eighteen months. Use of PTH is limited by high cost.

Strontium Ranelate

Treatment with strontium ranelate significantly reduces the risk of vertebral and non-vertebral fractures in osteoporotic patients, irrespective of the presence of a fracture or age. It both increases deposition of new bone osteoblasts and reduces the resorption of bone by osteoclasts, working as a dual-action bone agent.

Recent concerns about cardiovascular safety have limited the use of strontium ranelate to cases of severe osteoporosis in patients at low risk of cardiovascular disease.

Denosumab

Denosumab (Xzeva, Prolia, Olimab) is a human monoclonal antibody. At a dose of 60 mg used subcutaneously every six months, denosumab significantly reduces the risk of vertebral, non-vertebral and hip fractures and is safe and well tolerated. It is used when there is osteoporosis with a high risk of fracture or when there is intolerance to other therapies.

10

Heart and Cardiovascular System

'You've a good heart. Sometimes that's enough to see you safe wherever you go. But mostly, it's not.'

—Neil Gaiman

My mum's side of the family suffers from high blood pressure. My aunt, my uncle and my mum have all been on blood-pressure medication. My aunt's case, in particular, has been an amazing revelation on what BP medication can do to a woman. We know our BP fluctuates all through the day and even a small moment of anxiety could cause it to increase. Once you start BP medication, you are told not to stop it. However, over time it causes complications and some side effects. In my aunt's case, it was severe breathlessness until her medication was changed; however, the breathlessness never really went back to being under control.

I have worked with clients with whom we implement a diet and lifestyle change. Exercise, especially walking, helps, since if you are overweight, a reduction in weight will have a positive impact on your BP. You should closely monitor your BP and lipids to see how they are being impacted before a decision is taken to stop medication. But yes, good heart and cardiovascular health can be supported with a sound diet and lifestyle.

Shonali Sabherwal

My mother had a strong family history of heart disease. Her father died at the age of fifty-two and her younger brother, at forty-five years, suddenly and without warning, suffered a massive heart attack. She was a doctor with the most beautiful temperament, loved by every patient. She led the most perfect lifestyle with her diet and exercise routine. She was not yet menopausal in her fifties, though she would often voice concerns about her health, her looks and above all, her mental health when menopause would inevitably happen. Then, at fifty-five, she suddenly started experiencing breathlessness while climbing stairs. An angiogram found multiple blocks in her coronary vessels. She immediately underwent a coronary bypass, in which four blocks were found and corrected. At that time, twenty-five years ago, estrogen was believed to have a role in protecting the heart and its blood supply due to the fact that, prior to menopause, ischemic heart disease (IHD), where the blood supply to the heart is compromised, was far more common in men than in women. So, I started her on hormone therapy for heart protection, which she used happily for all its health and cosmetic benefits. Then came the results of an arm of the Women's Health Initiative (WHI) study that included older women using hormones for heart protection. The results concluded that the increased risk of stroke and breast cancer did not justify the treatment in spite of the significant reduction in fractures and colon cancer in this group. So, we stopped the MHT and she then used phytoestrogens for over ten years. Fifteen years later, she underwent an angiogram which found the repaired vessels in perfect condition. This I attribute largely to the brilliant work of the cardiac surgeon, but at least, and in significant part, to her lifestyle, her temperament and to the effect of estrogen use during those few years. It was for me a lesson in medicine regarding the important interplay of diet, lifestyle, emotions and medical treatment.

Nozer Sheriar

Women and Matters of the Heart

Estrogen seems to give women a clear cardiovascular advantage over men during their reproductive years. They have significantly lower risk of coronary artery disease and blockages in the vessels that give the heart muscle its blood supply, during their early lives. However, as estrogen levels fall in the perimenopause, women lose this hormonal advantage that protects the heart and its blood vessels, and the incidence of heart attacks soon equals that in men.

Cardiovascular disease becomes an important cause of serious illness, ICU admissions and death in post-menopausal women. Major primary prevention measures are to give up smoking, weight loss and weight control, BP reduction, regular aerobic exercise and correction and control of diabetes and lipid profile.

Interestingly, primary prevention strategies that are effective in men, such as the use of aspirin and statins to reduce abnormal cholesterol levels, do not seem to give the same protective effect for coronary heart disease (CHD), cardiovascular mortality or all-cause mortality in women.

What Types of Heart Disease Afflict Perimenopausal Women?

Cardiovascular disease (CVD) is the name for the group of disorders of the heart and blood vessels. While CHD dominates in perimenopausal women, they may manifest any of the entire range of cardiac conditions listed below:

- **Coronary heart disease** which we refer to as a heart attack.
- **Hypertension** which is high blood pressure (BP).
- **Congestive cardiac failure** which we term as heart failure.
- **Cerebrovascular disease** which presents as a stroke.
- **Cardiomyopathies** where there is an enlarged heart.
- **Peripheral vascular disease** which afflicts the distal blood vessels.

Each of these conditions has different predisposing factors, presentations and consequences. Since the presenting symptoms in early CVD, such as anxiety, weakness, fatigue, palpitations and sweating, could also be those of perimenopause, diagnosis may be delayed. As we know that perimenopausal women lose their cardioprotective privilege, it is important to consider the possibility of cardiac conditions for these symptoms, investigate them with an ECG and 2D echo and involve a specialist physician in your medical care.

How Do You Determine Your Risk of Developing CVD?

In general, cardiovascular disease will happen because of an accumulation of oxidized fat in blood vessels that eventually calcifies. Here are the factors associated with an increased risk for cardiovascular disease, particularly CHD, as outlined by Christiane Northrup:

- You are a habitual smoker.
- You have a strong family history of heart disease, especially before the age of sixty.
- Your bad cholesterol, LDL, is high and greater than 130 mg/dl.
- Your good cholesterol, HDL, is low and less than 46 mg/dl.
- You have high triglycerides, greater than 150 mg/dl.
- You have high BP, greater than 130/85 mm Hg.
- You have high levels of the amino acid homocysteine.
- You are obese with a BMI greater than 25.
- You have an apple-shaped figure with a preponderance of body fat above the hip level.
- Your waist measures over 85 cm or 33.5 inches.
- You have periodontal dental disease.
- You have diabetes.
- You are sedentary and do not exercise.
- You have a history of significant clinical depression.

To this list we would add insulin resistance, this being a major contributor to heart disease in women. A sign to recognize insulin resistance without measuring insulin levels is acanthosis nigricans, which is the darkening and velvety thickening of the skin folds in the neck, armpit and groin.

When cells become insulin resistant, glucose is left in the bloodstream, which then sends a signal to the pancreas to make more insulin. This leads to high BP, fat deposition, abnormal cholesterol and triglyceride levels and a clogging up of arteries. Insulin in excess results in elevated blood sugar levels. The resultant inflammation affects the lining (endothelium) of blood vessels. The elevated blood sugars attach to the bad LDL cholesterol molecules, causing them to stick to blood vessel walls. High stress levels can independently trigger cortisol release, leading to fat gain around the abdomen and insulin resistance. Having said that, even thin women may be insulin resistant, stress and consumption of poor-quality carbohydrates having a lot to do with their condition.

What Is Atherosclerosis and How Does It Predispose One to CHD?

Atherosclerosis is a condition of hardening and thickening of the walls of the arteries that takes place over time as the bad cholesterol (LDL) gets absorbed by immune cells that are on the surface of the endothelial cells, causing fatty deposits in the arteries. This happens due to free radical damage caused by a poor-quality diet, dietary fats, toxins in the environment and stress. Over time, these deposits become plaques. Plaques have cholesterol crystals at the centre and restrict blood flow as they grow. When they ulcerate and break away, bits of clots and calcified tissue (embolus) start moving with the blood, reaching areas of the body where they can cut off blood flow. When the coronary vessels supplying the heart muscle are blocked by the process of embolism, it results in heart attacks and when cerebral vessels in the brain are blocked, in strokes.

What Is the Association of Venous Thromboembolism (VTE) with the Perimenopause?

Venous thrombosis is when clots form in blood vessels and embolism is when a part of the clot breaks off and travels to another location to block a smaller blood vessel. During the perimenopause, venous thromboembolism is an important adverse event, not because of the condition itself, but as a rare consequence of hormone therapy. The incidence of VTE, deep vein thrombosis, where the deep vessels in the lower limbs are blocked, or pulmonary embolism, where the vessels in the lungs are blocked, is estimated to be 1 to 2 cases per 1000 woman-years of MHT use.

The risk for serious venous thromboembolic events related to MHT is rare in low-risk women until sixty years, but then increases with age, having an association with obesity and thrombophilia, a condition in which the normal process of breaking down of clots by the body is compromised.

How Does Estrogen Impact Heart Disease?

As we have read, estrogen is important in any discussion of women and heart disease because women are more prone to heart disease after menopause, a difference attributed to the lack of estrogen. While estrogen is looked at as preventing heart disease in women during reproductive life by favourably impacting the lipid profile, excess estrogen in some women may lead to blood clots and fluid imbalances, thus actually contributing to certain varieties of heart disease. Hence, your doctor knows best whether you are a candidate for MHT and how much estrogen you need.

What we do know is that estrogen has a protective effect on blood vessels and helps dilate the coronary arteries that supply the heart muscle. It directly modifies and normalizes the function of the endothelium (the inner lining of blood vessels) and smooths the muscles in their wall. It favourably impacts the lipid profile, benefits the good HDL and decreases the retention of bad LDL by the coronary arteries.

This is the rationale behind the belief that hormone therapy has the potential to improve the cardiovascular risk profile through its beneficial effects on vascular function, lipid levels and blood sugars.

There is good evidence that estrogen therapy may be protective for the heart if started around the time of menopause, often referred to as the 'window of opportunity', while it may be harmful when started more than 10 years after menopause. In women less than 60 years old, who are recently menopausal and with no evidence of CVD, estrogen-alone therapy reduces CHD and all-cause mortality rates. The evidence for combined oral estrogen–progestogen therapy is less convincing, although studies have also shown combined therapy to be cardioprotective.

CVD is the leading cause of death in women. Interestingly recent research shows a consistent benefit for women starting MHT before sixty years of age and within ten years of menopause.

What Is Nitric Oxide and How Does It Affect Blood Vessels?

Your arteries are vessels that carry blood away from the heart to all the organs and tissues in the body. They are lined with endothelial cells and damage to this inner lining of blood vessels over time predisposes you to heart disease.

Nitric oxide is produced by the endothelial lining of every blood vessel, in response to healthy pleasures such as exercise, taking vitamins and antioxidants, laughing, meditating and having sex. It has been linked to creating good heart health:

Nitric oxide not only increases blood circulation, it's also an über neurotransmitter that balances the levels of all the other neurotransmitters, including serotonin, dopamine, and endorphin. Plus it also helps quell cellular inflammation, which is the root cause of most chronic degenerative diseases.[*]

Nitric oxide naturally increases serotonin, the feel-good hormone.

In addition to nitric oxide, the endothelial lining of blood vessels secretes anticoagulants, molecules that prevent blood clots, occlusion of coronary vessels, heart attacks and embolic strokes, as also pro-clotting proteins, which prevent bleeding or haemorrhagic strokes. Damage to endothelial lining leads to inadequate production of nitric oxide or overproduction of the pro-clotting factors. When this is associated with stress and subsequent cellular inflammation, there is an increased risk for heart attack or stroke.[†]

---

[*] Northrup, Christiane, *Wisdom of Menopause*, Bantam Books, 2008, pp. 328–29.
[†] Ibid. p. 580.

Snapshot on Lifestyle and Diet

In my chosen professional lineage, which is the Traditional Chinese Medicine perspective, the positive emotion of the heart is 'joy' and the negative emotion is 'grief'. Most of my clients, almost all women, that come to me for heart ailments, have the common thread of 'grief' running through their lives, so you can imagine the unresolved emotions that women deal with in their lives. Samuel Mann, in his book Healing Hypertension: A Revolutionary New Approach, *infers trauma as a culprit in hypertension. By a woman's perimenopausal years, and this is from where I stand, you have either 'arrived'—resolved all the traumas you have been through—or you are still carrying a lot of 'baggage', which means you need to start shedding this load. Anxiety, depression, anger, hate, jealousy, irritation and disappointment are negative emotions that will constrict blood vessels, thereby restricting flow of blood to your organs, depriving them of nutrients and oxygen. It's a good time to live your truth, speak your mind, voice your emotions and let go of resentments. Go back into your life and 'mend' your broken heart.*

Shonali Sabherwal

Besides matters of the heart, lifestyle and diet play an important role. We all know when you have high BP, the doctor's first recommendation is to cut back your salt intake. BP can also be helped by increasing potassium in your diet, that is, if your hypertension is linked to high levels of sodium. The diet section deals with a sound plan to maintain this balance and prevent deficiencies in potassium.

Lifestyle Recommendations

- Avoid diuretics.
- Do not over workout. Keep the time to an hour.
- Avoid pain medication and blood thinners unless medically indicated.
- Avoid laxatives.
- Combat your stress with yoga, meditation and pranayama.
- Heart disease has a lot to do with grief, so please address it.
- Just move. Do everything to exercise, workout and live and practise yoga.

Diet Recommendations

- Focus on your fibre, whole grains, lentils, legumes, vegetables, nuts, seeds and fruit.
- Change salt to sea salt, rock salt or Himalayan pink salt.
- Focus on essential fatty acids, found in fish oil for non-vegetarians and chia or flax seeds for vegetarians. Non-vegetarians should incorporate fish at least thrice a week.
- Include garlic, even if it is in a capsule form, since it helps lower BP.
- Green tea helps with its flavonoids and its antioxidant effects.
- Add bone broth for collagen that keeps your connective tissue healthy around the heart.

Supplementation for Heart Health

- Magnesium is known to be a muscle relaxer. It stabilizes electrical conduction in the cardiac muscle and aids in regulating blood pressure. It also assists insulin with glucose transportation to cells. Stress, processed foods, diuretics, cow's milk with phosphates and high fluoride levels interfere with its absorption.

- Calcium works in tandem with magnesium and governs every cell in your body plus the electrical system of the heart. The ratio of balance of calcium to magnesium is between 1:1 and 2:1.

- Antioxidants play a vital role in heart and blood vessel health:

  - Coenzyme Q10 (CoQ10) is necessary for cell health, directing proteins to the areas of the cells that need repair. Without them, cells cannot carry out their genetic programming for cellular functioning and restoration. CoQ10 is necessary to produce energy in the form of ATP, the molecular currency of energy exchange of the cells. CoQ10 gives the heart the energy it needs to function. It improves the ability of the heart to pump more effectively, reducing congestive heart failure and BP. It also impacts cell membranes and has a role in the formation of collagen and elastin that make up the connective tissue in skin, muscle and blood-vessel walls.

  - Carotenoids present in foods like peppers (red and yellow), carrots, red pumpkin and the colours in fruits, have a positive impact on heart disease. Carotenoids such as beta carotene reduce free radical damage in the heart and blood vessels and prevent the bad lipoprotein (LDL) from being oxidized.

o Vitamin E keeps blood vessels slippery, reducing blood clots. It also benefits arrythmia (irregular heart rate) and cardiomyopathy (an enlarged heart).

o Tocotrienols are part of the vitamin E family. They play a role in all the major factors for coronary artery disease, particularly total cholesterol and LDL. They control an enzyme that controls the breakdown of LDL by your liver.

o Selenium used in a dose of 50–200 mcg per day decreases damage caused by free radicals in blood vessel walls.

o Proanthyocyanidins are in the class of foods known as flavonoids. CVD risk is inversely proportional to flavonoid intake. They are derived from grape seeds or pine bark. They are quickly absorbed into the bloodstream, help regenerate the body's levels of vitamin E and prevent oxidation of LDL cholesterol by free radicals. The usual dose is 40–120 mg/day.

o Alpha-Lipoic Acid (ALA) is an antioxidant that stands against free-radicals damage in every part of the cell. It preserves intracellular levels of vitamins C and E and is helpful in metabolizing insulin. It improves blood flow to both nerves and skin. The usual dose is 50–200 mg/day.

o Vitamin C is an antioxidant that helps protect the endothelial lining of your blood vessels and aids in the absorption of calcium and magnesium, the key minerals for heart health. If you have a sensitive stomach, use the ascorbate form. The recommended dose is 1000 mg/day.

- ○ Vitamin D deficiency has been associated with a host of health issues, but in heart health it impacts hypertension, several types of vascular diseases and heart failure. The recommended dose is 2000–5000 IU/day or 60,000 IU/month.

- ○ Folic acid is the antidote for high homocysteine levels, which increase the risk of clotting in blood vessels. Individuals with the highest homocysteine levels also have the lowest levels of folic acid, B6 and B12.

- ○ Niacin is a naturally occurring blood thinner that helps increase the good cholesterol (HDL), reducing inflammation and arterial constrictions. Niacin works by keeping the liver from eliminating HDL.

- ○ The usual doses of B vitamins are: 40–80 mg/day of vitamin B6, 20–50 mg/day of niacin, 20 mcg/day of vitamin B12 and 400–1000 mcg/day of folic acid. It is always better to take these together as an entire B complex preparation.

Medical Aspects of Heart and Vascular Disease in the Perimenopause

Apart from reduced estrogen levels, menopause also adds to other risk factors, including changes in body-fat distribution, abnormal blood sugar and lipid levels, increased blood pressure, increased sympathetic tone and inflammation in blood vessels. All women in the perimenopause should have periodic measurement of blood pressure and lipids (LDL, HDL, total cholesterol levels and triglycerides). Appropriate pharmacotherapy should be initiated when indicated. The use of low-dose aspirin is recommended in perimenopausal women at high risk of coronary heart disease.

We know that there is a window of opportunity in early menopause when cardiovascular harm can be avoided, and benefits achieved. While the baseline risk of coronary heart disease and stroke for women around menopausal age varies from one woman to another, according to the presence of multiple risk factors, MHT with estrogen alone is associated with no or reduced risk of coronary heart disease, while MHT with estrogen, with progestogen added for endometrial protection is associated with either a minimal or no increase in the risk of coronary heart disease.

Understanding Cardiovascular Risks of MHT

In women with high triglycerides (>400 mg/dL), obesity, a history of deep vein thrombosis and tobacco use, the non-oral route of MHT should be preferred, with use of transdermal estrogen as a patch or gel. The more natural progestogens with neutral effects on glucose metabolism, such as micronized progesterone or dydrogesterone, rather than synthetic progestogens, should be used for women with a uterus.

Venous thrombosis or clots in blood vessels increase with age and in the presence of other risk factors, including rare congenital or acquired thrombophilic disorders with a deficiency of anti-clotting factors such as proteins C and S and anti-thrombin III. A careful assessment of personal and family history of VTE is essential before prescribing MHT. The risk of venous thromboembolic events increases with oral MHT, but the absolute risk is rare below the age of sixty and in women with a normal BMI. The choice of hormones is important, with synthetic progestogens, such as medroxyprogesterone acetate, avoided due to increased risk. Although the incidence of VTE seems less frequent among Asian women, the possible risk must not be ignored.

11

Mental and Emotional Health

'*Keeping up the appearance of having all your marbles is hard work, but important.*'

—Sara Gruen

I lost a friend today; she jumped off the eighteenth floor. There were warning signs, but it was difficult for those around to babysit an adult. Yes, she was depressed and had been on antidepressants for a while. Her husband had told me a year ago that the downturn in her health started post menopause. He was bereft, as he didn't know how to help her. Nonetheless, he did try very hard, was extremely supportive and perhaps did not see this coming. As mentioned earlier, if you have not resolved your emotional baggage of your twenties and thirties, chances are they will manifest in your pre-menopausal and menopausal years. After our grief at the suicide, another friend and I vowed to reach out and meet more often and be there for each other in times of difficulty and need.

Shonali Sabherwal

L came to me five years ago when she was forty-five years old. She had been having delayed periods over many months, followed by no periods for three months with an FSH level of 27. This I treated with cyclic progesterone each month. She also complained of severe pre-menstrual symptoms (PMS), particularly breast tenderness, swelling and pain that started many days before her periods for which I prescribed evening primrose oil. A year later, she came with menopausal complaints of night sweats, bloating, breast tenderness and mood swings ranging from irritability to depression. Her FSH levels were now 116, she had multiple uterine fibroids and a mammogram showed multiple breast cysts.

L's preference was to avoid hormone therapy and with the dominant PMS-like breast symptoms I too favoured alternatives. She was advised a combination of lifestyle changes, suitable diet, evening primrose oil, local vaginal estrogens and soya-based naturally sourced estrogens of plant origin, called isoflavones. She has been well since then and has continued her treatment these last four years. Working with women has taught me what medical texts did not. PMS-like symptoms start dominating the hormonal situation for many women in their late thirties. They start before the period but gradually spread to most of the cycle, finally reaching a crescendo at menopause. Hormones do different things, physical and emotional, for different women and we have to recognize, acknowledge and factor this in when caring for them.

Nozer Sheriar

Why Do Mood Swings Tend to Dominate the Perimenopause?

Poonam would call me every day from Canada because she was feeling low and depressed. She wanted to reach out and unload all the time. As a practitioner in the field of health and wellbeing, the one thing you have to have is a lot of compassion; you can never turn off that tap and this is the way I dealt with her. I knew she needed to vent, so I let her. Much later, she took HRT and it proved to be extremely successful for her. But I still remember her telling me in those early days: 'I just don't want to get out of bed. Not only do my bones hurt, but so does my mind.' I never quite knew how that felt, but many women who describe their brains during these years, say that their brains are 'fried'. It is often the family that surrounds women that needs a lot of the support, to help them see them through this time.

Shonali Sabherwal

The emotional symptoms of the perimenopause are reflected early on in PMS symptoms that we don't give much significance to at the time. It is like PMS, only amped up, with crying jags, happy happies and cranky crankies. Your brain starts changing and, as Christiane Northrup says, since the changes in estrogen and progesterone affect the areas of your brain that make you irritable, anxious and emotionally volatile. While our beliefs and our culture leads us to believe that women's mood swings are simply the result of raging hormones, the repeated episodes of stress due to relationships, children and job situations that make you feel angry about or powerless over, may be behind many of the dramatic change.*

Is There a Link between PMS and the Perimenopause?

Your PMS years are a great indicator of what is to come in the midlife. It is estimated that 27 per cent of all women who experience agitation and depression during their periods and 36 per cent of all women who experience premenstrual depression will be very sensitive to the hormonal changes that occur at menopause.

PMS increases stress and stress increases cortisol levels. Cortisol is the hormone primarily released by the adrenal glands in response to feelings of fear, danger or even a sense of competition. When in excess, it can promote feelings of irritability, anger and depression, symptoms that can be common to both PMS and perimenopause. If you reach levels of exhaustion, cortisol is pushed again.

---

* Northrup, Christiane, *Wisdom of Menopause*, Bantam Books, 2008, p. 38.

The author Caroline Myss explains in *The Creation of Health* how stress impacts your life through her work on cancers.

> Think of yourself as a bulb full of energy where you expend a certain amount on day-to-day life activities such as working, exercising and bathing and another amount on thinking, ideating and mental activities. This uses up say 60% of your so called voltage. Now you get stressed and start overthinking and worrying and this starts eating away at the remaining 40%. When you are depressed, not only are you pushing cortisol, but also you have also exceeded the balance voltage or watts left in your bulb. Now you start eating away at cellular energy, the energy in your cells. This causes cells to also mutate and this may predispose and lead to cancers.[*]

Since cortisol and progesterone compete for common receptors in the cells, cortisol impairs progesterone activity, increasing estrogen and leading to estrogen dominance. High cortisol levels also impact your blood-sugar levels. In macrobiotics it is said that yin (sugar) craves more yin (sugar), so high blood-sugar levels mean you will start looking for something sugary and therefore gain weight. This is a vicious circle—once blood sugar levels are imbalanced, they will cause more cortisol to be released, which then causes craving for more calories.

Another hormone called prolactin, the hormone that is elevated when women are breastfeeding, is also elevated in

---

[*] Myss, Caroline and Shealy, C. Norman, *The Creation of Health*, Penguin Random House.

many women under constant stress. Hypothyroidism can also cause raised prolactin levels, which then results in in menstrual disturbance by interfering with the normal production of estrogen and progesterone. Shonali dealt with high levels of prolactin when under stress. A lot of inversion with yoga asanas really helped her along with her practice of meditation.

How Do You Cope with Sleep Disturbance in Menopause?

Much research has been conducted on sleep and we know how much the lack of a good night's sleep can affect our next day. This is especially true when you are dealing with fluctuating hormones and other issues during the perimenopause. While the tendency of the body is to go into a sleep-deprivation mode, these changes are speed breakers that must be navigated carefully. Shonali finds that the need for a good night's sleep in terms of hours has actually increased with age. Maybe it's because she exercises much harder than she used to and gets more tired, but two things have definitely changed: first, the number of hours of sleep she needs, which is precisely 7.5 hours; and second, the quality of her sleep has actually improved, and she sleeps right through the night. Being in the profession she is and thus highly in tune with her body, she finds that she sleeps well if she has eaten right and there have been no sugars in her diet that day.

So, if you suffer from insomnia, rectifying your eating and drinking habits is a must. If you have insomnia, then the midlife transition does become more difficult. It will decrease the levels of corticosteroids and catecholamines, which are stress hormones that can, in due course of time, throw off your hormonal balance, subsequently impacting the immune system. We all know that it is only during sleep that your mental and physical energy is renewed. Sleep also helps maintain a positive body weight.

Snapshot on Lifestyle and Diet

Lifestyle Recommendations

- Avoid caffeine post 5 p.m.
- Add strength or cardio workout.
- Eat whole grain, brown rice or millet, for two meals a day (especially dinner).
- Eliminate sugar.
- Dim the lights post 6 p.m. (this is one trick that has worked for Shonali for many years now).
- Stick to a sleep schedule around the same time every night, usually 10 p.m.
- Do not watch TV in the bedroom. The bedroom is for sleep and sex.
- Make sure you have a comfortable mattress and a good pillow.
- Avoid a heavy meal at dinner.
- Avoid tobacco.
- Avoid dairy.
- Keep your phone, computer and tablet away.
- Avoid arguments with your spouse, partner or anyone you are living with.

Diet Recommendations

A good diet such as the one outlined in the next section of this book and a good dose of sleep will have the following impact on you:

- Stress reduction.
- Reduction in inflammation.
- Improved memory.
- Weight loss.
- Reduced depression.
- Improved concentration.
- Improved memory.
- Lower risk of heart disease and strokes.
- Positive glucose metabolism.
- Stronger immunity.
- Greater gut function.
- Increased longevity.
- Freedom from pain because it act as a natural painkiller.
- Increased creativity.

Medical Treatment for Mental Health Issues

Hot flashes are the most common reason for sleep deprivation.

- MHT is the most effective treatment.
- Use cooler bedding. Avoid memory-foam mattresses as they make the body retain heat—stick to cotton mattresses.

Use cooling mattress pads and temperature-controlled mattresses that help with regulation of body heat.

- Maintain a sleep diary to assess sleep in detail.
- If you experience insomnia, you should be evaluated for medical or psychiatric causes, which if present should be treated.
- In case of suspected neurological or breathing disorders, get referred to specialists.

- Modify lifestyle; but if this difficult, then hypnotics such as zolpidem or benzodiazepines such as alprazolam, diazepam and lorazepam may be used in the short term, but only under medical supervision.
- Supplement with melatonin, which is a hormone secreted by the brain's pineal gland in response to darkness and released just before you sleep. You can safely supplement with up to 3 mg before bedtime.

Why do women grapple with anger and depression in the perimenopause?

As an adolescent, my thoughts were less about things that were affecting me on a larger canvas and more about my body. I was concerned about my attractiveness to the opposite sex. I did not focus on the fact that I may have had unresolved anger issues towards my father for having two different sets of rules for my brother and me, just because I was a girl, or even that I came close to sexual abuse by a relative. I pushed these larger issues aside then; but they came back to bite me much later in life.

While I do not have kids, I know what I went through in my early thirties, when I wanted to have them. I also know that women who do go through reproduction are filled with a flurry of reproductive hormones that actually stimulate the opioid centres of the brain. When my friend, Puja, was pregnant with her daughter, Meera, she would say, 'Sho, I feel great, I could climb a mountain.' I also know how I felt when my estrogen levels were high and when I was most attracted to men and how it would change depending on which phase of my menstrual cycle I was in.

Now, hurtling towards menopause, all of this has changed. Not that I don't feel attractive any more, but things have taken a turning and my hormones have shifted gears to set me up for the next phase in my life. I learnt through years of Vipassana meditation that the anger in my life ultimately was only towards myself and this pushed me towards self-realization. My reactions to external situations are now more a catalyst for inner wisdom, as I ask myself, 'what do I need to learn from this situation?'

A friend has been going through anger issues for years, even before her menopause. She has everything in terms of a good family, kids, husband, no money troubles, but her anger is directed outward towards everyone. She has never been the same since she lost her mother, who was her main support in her life, to cancer. Despite having the infrastructure and people to help her execute her projects, she is always angry, irritated and upset. One day, we were on a flight together and she asked me what the one thing was about her that I found wrong. I said, 'your anger. You just don't know how to control it; it controls you.'

She knows this—she is a smart woman—but she still hasn't done anything about it. I worry about her; she already has thyroid, rheumatoid arthritis and I fear she may get into something more. But all I can do is be there for her when she needs me.

Shonali Sabherwal

Menopause affects different women differently, so it is hard to say how rare or common menopause anger is. Feeling irritability and anger can be a result of many factors during the perimenopause. The realities of ageing, the physical and emotional changes of this new phase of life and the stress of lost sleep and hot flashes may cause women to experience a gamut of unstable moods. The perimenopause is also the time when women, who spend their life bearing the burden of tolerance and understanding in relationships with partners, children, families, friends and colleagues, reach the end of their tether and respond and react with an often-justified push back. This is misconstrued as women being irritable, difficult and unreasonable.

Women have historically played second fiddle to men, and their problems have often been ignored or gone undiagnosed. That Shonali's friend who died by suicide was indeed going through depression has been confirmed, but looking back, she had already shown signs of undue stress that may have been overlooked for almost a decade. The crucial hormones at play under a situation like this are GnRH (gonadotropin-releasing hormones) produced in your hypothalamus, a centre in the brain. The same hormones that control your menstrual cycle also influence serotonin, a brain chemical that promotes feelings of wellbeing and happiness. When hormone levels drop, serotonin levels also fall, which contributes to increased irritability, anxiety and sadness. This makes women less able to cope with things they would have normally coped with well and hormonal dips can set off a depressive episode, especially for those who've gone through major depression in the past.

This is the time for women to reach out and ask for help and for families and friends to be understanding and

give them the space and the support which women have so
unconditionally given them all these years.

Why Are Some Women Happier and More Balanced in the Perimenopause?

> *I have gone through some miserable times. I have been depressed and thought I would never pull out of it. This lasted for ten years of my life. But maybe all my prayers steered me in the direction of vipassanā meditation (parasympathetic nervous system activation), exercise, spiritual readings of various people like Osho, J. Krishnamurthi, Pupul Jayankar and Ramesh Balsekar which gave me some hope that I am attached to a larger force than just my small emotions of anger and hostility; additionally, by becoming a macrobiotic counsellor, I was able to sort out my diet imbalances. With all these efforts, I stepped out of that dark box and only moved forward from there on. I attracted new situations and circumstances, gained the conviction to quit my marriage and chart out a new path to becoming the person I am.*
>
> *Shonali Sabherwal*

Happy people have been described as having a higher
vagal tone, which simply means that their parasympathetic
nervous system (PNS) is more activated. This also
indicates their resilience to stressful situations. This part
of the autonomous nervous system is responsible for rest,
relaxation and conserving the energy in your body. Unhappy

people keep revving up their sympathetic nervous system (SNS), which helps the body cope with outside influences by causing a fight or flight response, the exact opposite of what the parasympathetic nervous system helps you do. By the time you head towards menopause, you are either holding on to your past and your 'tribal conditioning', which is what your parents passed on to you (negative or positive), or you have worked it all out, maybe gone to a counsellor or a psychologist or worked out your traumas through meditation, yoga, pranayama or some other tool. External incidents might disturb you and stir some residual anger, but they will pass. They will not cause you to go into a funk and, by this, I mean spiral downwards into a depression.

Immunity, strong or weak, is a direct result of the balance between the PNS and the SNS. Your T cells, involved in cell-mediated immunity (thymus), B cells, involved in antibody-mediated immunity (bone marrow or bursa derived), and red and white blood cells (bone marrow) are all triggered by the autonomous nervous system. A stressful life happens when your cortisol levels are always elevated, you are on a nutritionally deficient diet, you have a weak gut (with little absorption of nutrients) and a weakened adrenal function. You will have to address all the above factors to get you to be among the 'happy people'.

Why Does Dementia Occur More Frequently among Women?

The core mental functions are memory, communication and language, ability to focus and pay attention, reasoning and judgement, activities of daily living and visual perception.

Impairment of any two of these is suggestive of dementia. Many dementias are progressive, and an early diagnosis allows one to get the maximum benefit from available treatments and provides an opportunity to plan for the future.

Estrogen stimulates energy production, supports the immune system and has anti-inflammatory properties, so when it goes away there is a cost. According to Lisa Mosconi, an associate professor of neuroscience, '. . . estrogen keeps the brain young and juicy and active. As estrogen levels decrease, you lose a layer of protection and your brain can suffer.'

Mosconi's study looked at hundreds of brain scans of men and women. Men and younger women don't seem to show decline. Men, she says, don't show much neuron loss or build-up of plaques between neurons that are linked to the disease. Mosconi has found that brain energy decreases by up to 40 per cent on average during peri and early menopause, and women in this group have more Alzheimer's plaques than men of similar age or younger women. Of course, these changes are not found in everybody, and they are not found to the same degree in everybody.

It is important to note that menopause does not cause Alzheimer's. However, if you have a genetic predisposition to Alzheimer's, then during menopause, your brain can become less resilient and less able to slow the development of Alzheimer's plaques. With a clear link between estrogen levels and brain health, it makes sense to look at estrogen replacement therapy as an option for fighting cognitive decline. New studies are finding that starting ERT closer to menopause might help fight cognitive (mental and intellectual) decline. A cluster of lifestyle changes can also help reduce your risk of cognitive decline, lower risk of heart disease and also help alleviate other symptoms of menopause. Mosconi recommends a role for a Mediterranean diet that has lots of fibre that helps regulate estrogen levels. It includes vegetables, fruit, whole grains and legumes, with moderate amounts of fish and olive oil and limited meat and dairy. It is believed that eating this way can help lower your risk of heart disease, diabetes, hot flashes, cancer and dementia.

Snapshot on Lifestyle and Diet

Lifestyle Recommendations

- Make sure you have a workout protocol in place, whatever it may be since it releases endorphins, the feel-good hormones.
- Maintain the regularity of your mealtimes and eat at regular intervals.
- Engage in some form of activity to combat stress, like meditation, deep breathing or pranayama.
- Reset and rejuvenate by catching a good 7–8 hours of sleep and make up for it if you don't.
- Engage in an activity that keeps you connected to a group, since the team spirit of a group that you meet a couple of times a week always helps.
- Hang out with friends and, more importantly, reach out.
- Use a therapist to air your thoughts and feelings and get an impartial opinion.
- Try and come off anti-depressants, unless a specialist says you absolutely need them.

Diet Recommendations

- Quit refined sugar and refined foods and avoid artificial sweeteners.
- Keeping your blood-sugar levels stable is the key to combat any sort of a low. It keeps you clear of any brain fog or heightened state of mind.
- Minimize alcohol and drugs.
- Always stay hydrated.
- Minimize colas and sodas since they have caffeine and sugars or sugar derivatives, which worsen the situation.
- Include a whole grain in two meals since it helps keep the blood sugars stable. Focus on a high-fibre diet as outlined in the diet section.
- Use sweet potato and starchy foods as a snack early in the evening.
- Include good quality protein since it keeps you satiated and less cranky.
- Include good quality fats from foods. Keep trans fats and saturated fats at bay.
- Keep the gut flora balanced and the gut moving with fermented foods. The gut and brain have a deep connection since any inflammation in the gut will affect the brain.
- Take breaks and do some candle gazing.
- According to traditional Chinese medicine, the liver is the house of anger, your heart, of grief and your lungs, of depression. So please keep your liver happy by including greens, especially barley grass and spirulina, and pay attention to your heart and your lungs by practising healthy breathing techniques.

Supplements for Mental Health

- Include magnesium glycinate, which is a muscle relaxant.
- Vitamin B6 really helps by benefiting prolactin levels.
- Include curcumin, since it has a role in reducing inflammation.

Medical Treatment for Mental Health Issues

With menopause there is a window of vulnerability that makes some women more sensitive to the hormone shifts that occur, putting them at greater risk of mental-health issues. Many women are able to identify and describe their sources of tension and symptoms of stress, but may still find it difficult to take time for themselves. Emotional health during perimenopause requires a balance between self-nurturing, the obligations of work and caring for others. Recognizing a problem is the first step to finding ways to cope. Although many stressors cannot be altered, coping skills can enable you to meet life challenges and create a renewed sense of self confidence, balance and harmony.

It is important for a woman and her doctor to decide whether she is just feeling stressed or blue or whether she is clinically depressed. It is important for a woman to seek professional help and for her doctor to be attentive to her complaints and make a clinical judgement.

Major depression is a condition associated with a chemical imbalance in the brain. The changing hormones during perimenopause can be associated with that imbalance.

Depression is marked by the following symptoms:

- Prolonged tiredness.
- Low energy.

- Loss of interest in normal activities.
- Sadness and irritability.
- Sleep disturbances.
- Agitation.
- Weight changes.
- Decreased sex drive.

Although most people will experience these symptoms from time to time, they have to last for more than two weeks to suggest major depression.

Depression across the menopause has a multifactorial aetiology. There are predictive factors that include:

- Previous depressive episodes such as PMS and/or postpartum depression.
- Menopausal symptoms, especially hot flashes, nocturnal sweating and insomnia.
- Menopause not treated with MHT.
- Major existential stress.
- Elevated body-mass index.
- Low socioeconomic level and ethnicity.

Post-menopausal depression is more severe, has a more insidious course, is more resistant to conventional antidepressants in comparison with pre-menopausal women. It has better outcomes when antidepressants are combined with MHT.

The Modified Depression Anxiety Stress Scale

The DASS scale was designed and standardized as a self-administered scale to assess the three related negative emotional states of depression, anxiety and tension/stress. You can use this scale to gain an objective insight into your situation, whether you are suffering mental or emotional anguish and understand when to seek professional help.

Based on this scale we have created a self-test with simple situational experiences to evaluate your emotional situation. You assign a score from zero to three, with zero being does not apply to me and three being does apply to me very much or most of the time. The total score is a sum of the scores (number) you assign to each answer. There are no right or wrong answers.

Which of the following feelings or emotions apply to you at this time?

Your thoughts and experiences	0	1	2	3
I am charged up and unable to wind down				
I experience dryness in my mouth				
I do not feel any positive feelings				
I find difficulty in breathing when stressed				
I find it difficult to want to do things				
I tend to overreact to small things				
I find my hands trembling with nervousness				
I feel wound up a bundle of nerves				
I worry that I may panic and make a fool of myself				
I feel gloomy with nothing to look forward to				
I find myself easily getting riled up and agitated				
I just cannot find it in me to unwind and relax				
I feel low and blue and down hearted				
I am intolerant to anything that comes in my way				
I am often in a state of utter panic				

I am unable to feel enthusiastic about anything				
I feel unworthy with low self confidence				
I feel very touchy about the smallest things				
I feel my heart racing even when I am resting				
I am scared about the smallest things for no reason				
I feel life is pointless and meaningless				

Interpretation of scoring of symptoms to determine emotional state

	Normal	Mild	Moderate	Severe	Extremely Severe
Anxiety	0-2	3-4	5-7	7-9	10+
Depression	0-4	5-6	7-9	10-13	14+
Stress	0-7	8-9	10-12	13-16	17+

Forgetfulness, Cognitive Symptoms and Dementia

Forgetfulness, trouble concentrating, and other cognitive (mental and intellectual) symptoms are common during midlife. During the menopausal transition, many women experience transient cognitive impairment, which is usually of small magnitude. There is likely to be no persisting effect of the natural menopause on memory or other cognitive functions.

With surgical menopause where the transition is abrupt and which occurs at an earlier age, estrogen therapy has short-term cognitive benefit when initiated at the time of removal of the ovaries.

Medical strategies to prevent dementia:

- MHT within five years of menopause reduces the risk for developing Alzheimer's disease in later life by 30 per cent.
- Diets high in Omega 3 fatty acids, especially docosahexaenoic acid (DHA), reduce the risk of developing dementia by 50 per cent.
- Women with higher levels of baseline physical activity are less likely to develop cognitive decline.
- Learning new skills helps build cognitive reserve and staves off dementia.
- Consuming antioxidants such as vitamin E will help the body reduce free radical associated changes.

Low Mood and Anxiety

The low mood and anxiety that arises as a result of menopause can be alleviated by MHT. The role of counselling and cognitive behavioural therapy in such situations cannot be overstressed.

Possible treatments for menopause-related anxiety include:

- MHTs.
- Antidepressants—SSRIs or SNRIs.
- Psychotherapy.
- Supplements such as pyridoxine for better mood.

Major Depression

MHT has been reported to improve depressive symptoms in post-menopausal women. A trial of systemic estrogen therapy is recommended for women with symptoms of depression and other bothersome menopause symptoms. This may be recommended for women who are unable or unwilling to take antidepressants.

Menopausal women and their doctors should seek specialist psychiatrist referral in situations of major depression. The use of SSRIs such as fluoxetine, paroxetine or sertraline or SNRIs such as duloxetine or vanafaxine for managing depression could be combined with MHT and cognitive-behavioural psychotherapy.

This combination of antidepressants with MHT seems to offer the best therapeutic potential in terms of effectiveness and rapidity of improvement.

12

Cancers in Perimenopause

'You never know how strong you are until being strong is the only choice you have.'

—Cayla Mills

Supriya came to me after her breast cancer had spread to her brain and liver. This is her story in her own words:

I received a stage-IV breast cancer diagnosis for which I underwent chemotherapy and radiation. Initially, I responded well to treatment but, after a short while, there was disease progression. Despite being treated with the best medicines, I felt really helpless. I wanted to be in control of my health and life. Doctors think it's okay to keep taking medicines indefinitely, but I wasn't comfortable with that. I had been following Shonali on social media for a while and found her in-depth knowledge of using nutrition to reverse illness simply incredible. I started consulting with Shonali soon after the scans detected progression. My diet changed completely, and I followed her instructions strictly on what, how and when to eat. Just 3–4 months later, my scans turned out to be excellent. Most of the metastatic lesions were no longer there. I had expected results, but this was beyond anything I could have imagined. I could feel the difference in my digestion, energy, skin and hair health. I was very happy to be feeling and looking good. I have gained a wealth of knowledge regarding food and nutrition and that has changed how my entire family eats. I feel a lot more empowered about my health. I can see myself going off cancer medication in the near future and I am really looking forward to that.

Shonali Sabherwal

N has been my patient for twenty-four years, since when she was just twenty-seven years old, during which time she has had three great kids—twenty-three, fourteen and twelve years old. Over the years, she has been a model patient, coming in for regular health check-ups, Pap smears, ultrasounds, mammograms and bone-density studies. She had heavy periods, which we managed with oral-contraceptive pills and large uterine fibroids, for which we avoided surgery. She started her perimenopause when she was forty-five with FSH levels of 56 but went on with irregular periods for the next four years. Her routine annual ultrasound this year unexpectedly showed a large 8 cm growth in her right ovary with increased blood flow. Within less than a week she underwent an extended hysterectomy, with the removal of both ovaries and multiple lymph nodes. Histology confirmed an ovarian cancer called a granulosa cell tumour. The nodes were negative for any spread. Thankfully, this meant that the surgery was her cure and there was no need for chemotherapy. That her husband was a most sensitive and supportive partner made all the difference as they went through this trying time together. Since then, her main complaint has been vaginal dryness which we are managing with vaginal application of estrogen cream. N exemplifies for me the value of sincere screening in the early diagnosis and successful treatment of cancers in women. She also demonstrates that neither cancer nor its treatment can stop us from treating the symptoms of menopause.

Nozer Sheriar

Basics of Cancer: The Dreaded 'C' Word

Cancer occurs when cells multiply faster than normal with a disturbance in the process called apoptosis, the technical term for programmed cell death. This could take place due to various reasons that are compounded by diet, emotions, environmental factors, exposure to toxins causing free radical damage—anything that disrupts the environment within the cell. Programmed cell death is necessary for our health to be maintained as our bodies renew themselves throughout our lives. Cancer is predisposed to or comes from an imbalance in our bodies and if we can somehow manage to correct the imbalance, we can minimize our risk, limit the disease and even improve our chances for a cure.

All cancer starts due to a change in your own cells, when cells start multiplying at an abnormal rate, not growing into the cells that they ought to be and instead becoming cancer cells that have lost the ability to differentiate. It is at this stage that the disease originates, as cancer cells escape the ability to follow the normal control that the body exerts on cells. As these cells grow and divide, they clump into a mass or masses which are called 'tumours'. As they then disperse from these tumours to other parts of the body, either directly or by the blood or the lymphatic system, the process of spread is called 'metastasis'.

Cancer cells are different from normal cells because they:

- Divide out of control.
- Avoid detection by the immune system.
- Ignore signals that tell them to stop dividing or tell them to die when they should.
- Are immature and do not develop into mature cells when they should.
- Can spread to other parts of the body through the blood or the lymphatic system.
- Grow into and damage tissue and organs.

Cancer cells have the same needs as normal cells—they need blood supply to bring in oxygen and nutrients to grow. So, they send signals to a tumour to grow, inducing increased blood supply and a network of new blood vessels (neovascularization), supporting their rapid growth and spread.

The word 'remission' is used when the cancer comes under control and there are no signs or symptoms of the disease. The goal of treatment is to induce and stay in the remission period as far as possible. When cancer comes back, it is referred to as a 'recurrence'. Even if a few cells are left behind after treatment, they could start up the same cancer initiation process as before. In some cases, treatment might stop being effective and in others, the cancer cells get resistant to treatment.

Gynaecological Cancers in India

In India, cancer is an important public health problem with over 8,00,000 new cases occurring every year. More than 80 per cent of cancers in women occur between the ages of thirty-five and sixty-five years, with the highest burden being during the perimenopause. The leading sites of cancer among women are related mainly to four organs: breast, cervix, body of the uterus and ovaries. These account for over 60 per cent of all cancers. This is both a problem and an opportunity, since attention to these through prevention, early detection and appropriate timely treatment offers possibility of success and survival like never before.

Breast Cancer

Breast cancer is the most common cancer among women worldwide and in India. It accounts for 28 per cent of cancers among women in India, with one in twenty-eight women likely to develop breast cancer in their lifetime.

Risk Factors for Breast Cancer

The midlife is the time when your chances of getting breast cancer are on the rise. This also happens to be the time generally associated with the cumulative risk of an unhealthy lifestyle and eating patterns.

The following risk factors should be considered:

- Over fifty years of age with risk increasing until eighty years of age.
- Early onset of menstruation, that is, before the age of twelve.
- Family history of breast cancer, in either a first-degree relative (mother, sister or daughter) or a second-degree relative (maternal or paternal grandmother or aunt).
- Late menopause, after fifty-five years.
- Giving birth to a first child after thirty years.
- No full-term pregnancies.
- Long-term hormone therapy.

Screening for and Early Diagnosis of Breast Cancer

A breast self-exam is a check-up you do at home to look for changes or problems in the breast tissue. While experts do not all agree about the benefits of breast self-exams, many feel that doing this is important for health. We consider this an important tool to ensure awareness and a personal commitment to be involved with one's own health. The best time to do a monthly self-breast exam is about three to five days after your period since your breasts are not tender or lumpy at this time. After menopause, do your exam on the same day every month.

How to Do a Self-Breast Examination (BSE)

1. Stand in front of the mirror. Examine both breasts, first by looking at the shape, contours, change in nipples or any dimples. Next, rest your palms on your hips and press firmly to flex your chest muscles. Left and right will not exactly match, few women's breasts do. Look for puckering, dimpling, changes, particularly on one side.

   Using the pads of your fingers, move around your breast in a circular motion, moving from the outside to the inside, including the armpit area, looking for lumps,

Figure 14: How to do a breast self-examination

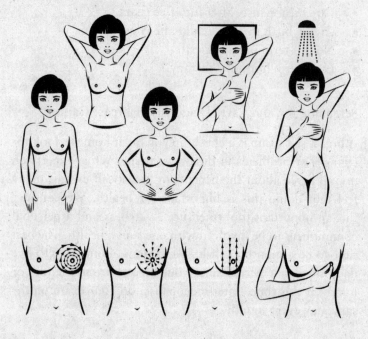

thickening or irregularity. Do this in the shower with soap so your fingers move smoothly over the breast.

2. Squeeze the nipples, checking for discharge and lumps.
3. Lying down, examine the breast tissue as it spreads out evenly along the chest wall. Place a pillow under your shoulder and your arm behind your head. Using your other hand, move the pads of your fingers around your breast gently in small circular motions covering the entire breast area and armpit. Use light and firm pressure.

Screening for Breast Disease

Let me share something here that happened to me a few years ago, when I was on an exercise regimen and had shed a lot of weight. Naturally, my breasts also lost some fat. One day, while feeling my breasts, I discovered a small lump on my right breast. I had my period coming up in a week and my annual examination coming up with Dr Nozer in two weeks; so I decided to go get a sonography of the breast done. The radiologist, Dr Varisht Hingorani, MD, a calm and amazing guy, said it didn't look like anything to worry about and suggested that I use an ice pack. It seemed to him this lump was inflamed considering I had been prodding a bit too much and that I should come back after my period to see where I stood. Was I nervous? No. I know what the mind-body connection is and how thoughts can really affect the body, so I walked around for two weeks with this blue-gel ice-pack stuck over one breast and absolutely forgot I even had this occurrence. My mother, of course, always playing the devil's advocate, was worried as hell and kept asking me what I would do if the dreaded C happened? I minimized phone calls with her for two weeks.

Two weeks later, after my period, I landed up at Dr Hingorani's clinic again and there was no lump. It had disappeared. Now, if this had been my sister, she would have panicked, gone for a mammogram, done many tests and even if this lump was just fatty tissue or some cyst that had come up, she would have had it surgically removed. This does not mean that you should not get lumps in the breast that you find checked. Of course, you should, as I did, but there is no need to panic, that's what I am trying to establish within this story. Not all lumps are malignant, and a woman could have many small cysts and lumps in her life that are just there because they form a part of your breast anatomy.

Shonali Sabherwal

Mammograms and Sonomammograms

Sonomammograms, mammograms and MRIs do not prevent breast cancer but assist in early diagnosis of disease. Treatment at an early stage has higher success and survival rates. A reasonable protocol for mammography is as follows:

- Women who do not have an increased risk of breast cancer should be offered a screening mammography starting at the age of forty years.

- Women aged between forty-five and fifty-four years should be screened annually.
- Women fifty-five years and older should transition to biennial screening or have the opportunity to continue screening annually.
- Women should continue screening mammography as long as their overall health is good and they have a life expectancy of ten years or longer.

While mammograms can be a wonderful tool to detect cancers, there is a caveat. Many women live with a condition called ductal carcinoma in situ (DCIS), a type of breast pathology that can often remain completely dormant for a woman's entire life. Many studies point to the fact that the incidence of DCIS has increased since 1980 and this accounts for a major portion of cancers picked up by a mammogram. However, the increase coincides with the widespread use of mammographic screening.

Like all early detection strategies, screening mammography involves trade-offs. To truly participate in the decision of whether or not to be screened, you need some quantification of its benefits and harms. In a study by Welch and Passow of 1000 US women aged fifty years who were screened annually for a decade, around three avoided a breast cancer death, half had at least one false alarm, and around ten were over diagnosed and treated needlessly. Understand these ranges so that you either to feel comfortable about their decision to pursue screening or to feel equally comfortable about their decision not to pursue screening.

Should You Test Yourself for the Breast Cancer Gene?

While 95 per cent of all breast cancers have little or nothing to do with genetics, 5 per cent are linked to two genes: BRCA1 and BRCA2. Women who inherit BRCA1 mutation have a higher risk of cancer compared to those with a BRCA2 mutation. They have a 56 per cent lifetime risk of breast cancer and an estimated 15 per cent risk of developing ovarian cancer by the age of seventy years of age. Angelina Jolie had the BRCA1 gene mutation, and chose to go through preventive breast cancer surgery, a double mastectomy. Media dubbed it as the 'Angelina Jolie Effect'. Granted, she had seen her mother going through it for ten years and therefore her chances were high of getting the cancer. However, when you piece the whole picture together it is safe to conclude that genetic testing for breast cancer is still incomplete and needs to be interpreted in context.

Does Estrogen Exposure Increase Risk of Developing Breast Cancer?

When comparing the hormone receptors of breast-cancer cells with the state of differentiation, it is discovered that a predominance of estrogen receptors correlates with less differentiated, more dangerous cancer cells; the presence of progesterone receptors correlates with cancer cells that are more differentiated and less dangerous. Estrogen activates a cancer promoting gene called Bcl-2, which slows apoptosis (cell death), while progesterone activates gene p53, which actually restores proper apoptosis. So, when we consider apoptosis and cell differentiation, we can conclude that estrogen is a promoter of breast cancer and progesterone is a protector.

Besides estrogen, breast-tissue growth can happen due to estrogen mimicking substances such as xenoestrogens. Early menstruation before twelve years of age, a diet that is not helping your insulin but causing insulin sensitivity, PCOS and women who have never been pregnant or have never lactated are all factors increasing risk. Diet affects your breast health a lot and should be completely taken into account. Progesterone may reduce the activity in the estrogen-receptor production in breast-cancer cells and decrease estrogen within them. Of course, this protection may be impacted and unavailable in progesterone-receptor-positive cancers.

Ultimately, creating good breast health is in your hands. Living with fear is a choice you have and make. Similarly, choosing happiness and an attitude to life and living healthy via diet, exercise, meditation, sleep, bodywork like massage or other therapies is entirely in your hands and something you have control over.

Cervical Cancer

How many women talk about their cervix? None. We all know it's a spot that our gynaecologist examines when we go for our pap smears and is the part that dilates to let our babies be born, but that is about as far as our knowledge goes. Nevertheless, it is an important area, albeit much neglected.

Your cervix is at the base of the uterus. It is the part that extends into your vagina; the same part a baby uses to exit the womb. It is like the neck of the uterus. It is narrow yet changes in size when labour begins to prepare for childbirth. It will change its shape, colour, position and size depending on your menstrual cycle and level of sexual arousal. Mine, Dr Nozer has told me during our usual conversations when he is palpitating my uterus and ovaries, is forwards with my uterus retroverted. Now you know, too!

Shonali Sabherwal

Cervical cancer is the fourth most common cancer worldwide for females, and the seventh most common cancer overall, with more than 5,27,000 new cases diagnosed annually. The peak age for developing cervical cancer is between thirty and thirty-five years and this declines steadily after this until a second peak in incidence in very old age. A majority of women are diagnosed in a late stage of this cancer, which is unfortunate, because this particular cancer gives the doctor adequate opportunity to intervene successfully years before progression.

When you visit your gynaecologist, a Pap smear, a smear or scraping of some tissue from the opening of the cervix is taken to detect cancerous or pre-cancerous cells in your cervix. An estimated eight out of ten women do not do routine Pap smears and this is unfortunate, since a Pap smear is perhaps the best test there is to detect early signs of cancer of the cervix. Regular Pap smears done annually will help you to detect abnormal growth in cells early and in the pre-cancerous phase, allowing prevention, halting progression or achieving a complete cure. Combining HPV testing with the Pap smear makes it even more effective.

Human Papilloma Virus (HPV) causes a viral infection. This virus has many types of viral strains. Of these, fourteen are identified as high-risk types. These include HPV 16 and 18 and are said to be responsible for almost all cervical cancers. Not only does this make testing for HPV an important part of screening, but if you are negative for a high-risk type of HPV and if your Pap smear is normal, you are considered low risk and may screen less frequently, once in four to five years and not annually, as recommended with traditional Pap smears. The HPV vaccine has a significant role in reducing the risk of cervical cancer. However, even if you have taken the HPV vaccine at a younger age, you should still get regular Pap smears since not all high-risk types are covered by the existing vaccines and no vaccine is infallible.

National screening programmes in many developed countries have led to a significant decrease in incidence of cervical cancer, with the incidence in women aged over forty-five years having declined significantly since the mid-1970s.

An abnormal Pap smear covers a spectrum of mild to severe dysplasia, where there are abnormal cells within the cervical epithelium. If you have an abnormal Pap smear, your doctor might recommend a procedure called colposcopy and if an abnormal area is seen, it is biopsied.

What Are the Symptoms of Cervical Cancer?

The earlier stages of disease are symptomless. The commonest complaint is abnormal discharge or bleeding, often experienced as bleeding after sex. There may be increased frequency of urination and pain while urinating and pelvic pain which might be a late symptom.

Are There Measures That May Help Prevent Cervical Cancer?

Vaccination and regular screening have the potential to actually prevent cervical cancer or detect and manage it in the pre-cancerous or early stages.

- Take the vaccine if between ages nine and twenty-six years.
- Practice safe sex, as HPV is sexually transmitted.
- Avoid smoking.
- Get regular and routine Pap smears.

Endometrial Cancer

Endometrial cancer, also called uterine cancer, is caused by unopposed estrogen stimulus that results in abnormal cell growth in the endometrial lining. The more periods you have, the more the endometrium is exposed to estrogen; so girls that start menstruating early or those women that hit menopause late are at risk, as are women who have never been pregnant.

Besides this unopposed estrogen stimulus with estrogen only HRT increases the risk, though this can be completely nullified by adding a progestogen. Excess body fat changes hormones and could be another factor. Women treated with tamoxifen after breast cancer are also likely to be more at risk of abnormal endometrial changes.

What Are the Symptoms of Endometrial Cancer?

You may have a previous history of irregular and delayed periods over time as a predisposing factor. Unscheduled bleeding between periods, heavy periods, vaginal bleeding after menopause has set in, bloody discharge from the vagina are some symptoms and pelvic pain might be a late symptom.

Are There Steps to Prevent Endometrial Cancer?

- Keep your weight under check at all times and exercise.
- Consider taking oral contraception pills or progestogen-only contraception such as progestogen-only pills, injections, hormonal intrauterine device and implants since these reduce your cancer risk.
- If you are on MHT using estrogen alone, do discuss the risks with your doctor.

Ovarian Cancer

A woman's lifetime risk of developing ovarian cancer is one in seventy-eight and her lifetime risk of dying from invasive ovarian cancer is one in 108. Ovarian cancer rates are highest in women aged between fifty-five and sixty-four years.

Ovarian cancer is the third most common cancer among women and the fifth leading cause of cancer-related death. Ovarian cancer generally goes undetected and by the time it is detected, it has already spread to other parts of the body. This local and remote metastasis has a very high mortality rate. Over 80 per cent of ovarian cancers are epithelial ovarian tumours from the surface cells, although ovarian cancers can arise from every part of the ovary, that is, the stroma and the germ cells, leading to far more varieties than other cancers.

The best way for a doctor to diagnose ovarian cancer is to palpate (that is feel the ovaries with the hand) during a pelvic exam or a pelvic ultrasound. Menopausal women have smaller ovaries that are not detectable with palpitation so the presence of a larger ovary in a menopausal woman can be a cause for concern.

What Are the Risk Factors for Ovarian Cancer?

- Fertility drugs without adequate supervision for extended periods.
- Genetic predisposition.
- Consumption of dairy products.
- Women who haven't had children, since pregnancy is a rest-phase for the ovaries.
- Older age.
- Presence of either the BRCA1 or the BRCA2 gene.
- Early or late menstruation.

What Are the Symptoms of Ovarian Cancer?

- Bloating.
- Pain and cramping
- Irregular bleeding during a menstrual cycle and changes in menstruation.
- Fatigue.
- A feeling of fullness or undigested food.
- Changes in bowel movements.

- Frequent need to urinate.
- Discomfort in pelvic region.
- Weight loss.

How Does One Lower the Risk of Ovarian Cancer?

- Using birth-control pills.
- Tubal ligation, where fallopian tubes are tied to prevent pregnancy.
- Oophorectomy (removal of the ovaries) or just removal of the tubes even when conserving ovaries at hysterectomy.
- Pregnancy and breastfeeding.
- Diet and exercise.

What Is the Significance of the Frequently Reported Ovarian Cysts?

It is important that you know that most times if you have cysts on your ovaries, they are completely normal. Enlarged cysts are common and very often not cancerous. At the start of each cycle, more than a few follicles will mature. One of these follicles will dominate and release its egg into the fallopian tube, leaving the rest to get reabsorbed or dissolve. Cysts are a normal phenomenon in the ovulation process in a woman's life and functional ovarian cysts can come up, grow large (up to 5 cm) and then vanish suddenly. Depending on the structure from which the cyst develops, they are classified as follicular cysts (from the follicle) or luteal cysts (from the corpus luteum). Functional cysts do not need surgical intervention, only observation until they disappear.

What Are Oophorectomies?

An oophorectomy is a surgical procedure to remove one or both of your ovaries. You should know about this because it is essential for your overall hormonal health to retain your ovaries wherever possible.

In some cases, however, there is no choice but to let them go. Oophorectomy is usually done in the following conditions:

- Ovarian cancer.
- A pus-filled abscess involving the ovary.
- Endometriotic cysts and severe endometriosis only if the ovary cannot be saved.
- Non-malignant ovarian cysts.
- Ovarian torsion (twisting of your ovary), although all efforts must be made to save the ovary.
- Reducing risk of breast and ovarian cancer in high-risk situations such as BRCA1 and 2 positives.

If you have not gone through menopause, then losing your ovaries will immediately put you into premature menopause. Even after menopause, ovaries still retain useful hormonal function so you may want to request conservative surgery and ovarian retention in endometriosis, benign ovarian cysts and torsion, although the final decision has to be that of the surgeon after you have a detailed conversation about alternatives.

Surgeons tend to recommend or perform an oophorectomy in women undergoing hysterectomy if they are aged over forty-five years, with the stated purpose of preventing ovarian cancers going ahead. The current practice is to save the ovaries since the risk of such cancers is small and the benefits of ovarian function far outweigh these risks. Sacrificing the ovaries increases your risk of CHD and stroke, increases chances of cognitive impairment and dementia, increases the risk of osteoporosis and hip fracture and predisposes to more depression and anxiety later in life. You should stand up for your ovaries and fight to keep them where possible.

Snapshot on Lifestyle and Diet

There are various reasons why cancers happen. Keeping our cellular structure healthy is of primary importance in prevention of cancer or if you have cancer. I have helped many women in both scenarios, and we have managed the cancer very well. I have worked with women who come from families with a history of cancer, women post-surgery, women undergoing radiation, women who are going through chemotherapy and those who have finished their chemotherapy cycles. In every case, the approach is to keep the blood condition (pH) in balance and assist women with their diet, lifestyle and emotional health.
Shonali Sabherwal

Lifestyle Recommendations

- Make yourself a priority.
- Make sure you have a set routine.

- Keep yourself oxygenated with exercise and breathing (pranayama).
- Let go of any grudges you may be holding on to.
- Take the assistance of a psychologist.
- Surround yourself with positive energy always.
- Surround yourself with green plants for extra oxygen.
- Use iron cookware, ceramic or stainless-steel utensils.
- For those on chemotherapy or undergoing treatment who do not feel like eating due to a change in taste or low appetite, remember you must eat even if it is smaller meals in a soup format or in small bowls, taking a few tablespoons at a time.
- As an anti-cancer approach, food has to be used as a medicine to help you.

Diet Recommendations

- Stay away from sugar (sugar derivatives), dairy, refined, processed and packaged foods.
- Change your salt to sea, rock or Himalayan pink salt.
- Change to cold-pressed oils since they do not cause free radical damage.
- Use fermented foods as they provide fresh nutrients and also feed the good gut bugs.
- Make sure you eat foods that are home cooked and focus on colourful vegetables, legumes, lean protein or plant-based protein, fruit, whole grains (millet and brown rice), seeds and nuts. Try staying more plant-based unless you are going through chemotherapy. Then a bone broth would help keep you strong.
- Indoles in cabbage, lycopene in tomatoes, allicin in garlic and immune boosters in sea vegetables are a new category of minor dietary constituents (MDC).

- Focus on carotenoids since these are free radical protectors. Bioflavonoids do the same by absorbing dangerous unpaired electrons. Both these stimulate the immune system and are found in citrus, whole grain, honey (manuka) and many plant foods.
- Cruciferous vegetables such as broccoli, brussels sprouts, cabbage and cauliflower have indoles and are protective in cancer. They also increase the body's production of glutathione peroxidase, which is one of the most important enzymes in the body.
- Mushrooms, rei-shi, shiitake and maitake are very potent anti-cancer foods.
- Maitake contains a polysaccharide called beta-glucan, which stimulates the immune system.
- Soybeans have substances that are protein inhibitors that quash tumour growth. They also have isoflavones and phytoestrogens, which appear to have potential anti-cancer properties.
- Have 2–3 green juices a day between meals with a carrot and avocado for good fats. Rotate greens by using different greens every week.
- Add spirulina (sea vegetable), particularly during chemotherapy, as it helps absorb its negative effects, or use a greens formula.

Health Foods That Can Help You

- Broccoli has folate, and spinach and leafy greens have vitamin E, which is a big help when it comes to cervical health.
- Grapefruit and tomatoes have lycopene, which helps those who have HPV infection.

- Red pumpkin (lal kaddu/bhopla) or any other coloured vegetable has beta carotene which converts to vitamin A and helps the immune system.
- Bell peppers are rich in vitamin C, as are citrus fruits. They help with immunity.

Supplements

- Up your vitamin C intake. Avoid during chemo or radiation as cancer cells are 'gluttons' for vitamin C, absorbing more than their fair share of it.
- Up your vitamin D if low.
- Up your zinc.
- Check selenium levels and if low, add it.
- Check magnesium levels and if low, add it.
- Take Co Q-10.
- Take a greens complex if greens run low in your diet.
- Add green tea or a green-tea supplement for catechins and epigallocatechin. This is also found in apples.
- Quercetin is a supplement found in kale, spinach, onions, apples and black tea.
- Add alpha-lipoic acid.
- Up your vitamin A.
- Add curcumin as an anti-inflammatory.
- Use garlic and ginger in foods.
- Add ellagic acid, found in cranberries, raspberries and other berries.
- Add anthoyacyanins, found in dark-coloured fruits (blueberries), vegetables, red onions and black sesame seeds
- Ginseng is known to help cancer patients. It has adaptogenic qualities (properties that help the body

cope with stress), boosts the central nervous system, is a blood-glucose regulator, has immune-stimulating effects, provides liver-cleansing protection and stimulation and is an anti-coagulant.

- Add a fish-oil supplement.
- All supplements should be managed by a healthcare provider.

Medical Management of Cancers in the Perimenopause

Management of Breast Cancer

The value of early diagnosis of breast cancer by self-examination, mammography, sonography or MRI cannot be overstressed since early-stage breast cancers have an excellent prognosis, with survival rates of well over 95 per cent. These drop to 30 per cent with distant spread.

Early-Stage Breast Cancer

Early-stage breast cancers are treated initially with surgery:

- Lumpectomy conserves the breast.
- Mastectomy involves the removal of the entire breast.
- Lymphadenectomy samples the lymph nodes in the axilla (armpit) and may be performed at the time of surgery depending on the type and extent of the tumour.

Both types of surgery may be followed by radiation therapy and chemotherapy:

- Chemotherapy for breast cancers with estrogen receptors (ER), progesterone receptors and human epidermal growth factor receptor 2 (HER 2).
- Endocrine therapy specifically for hormone-receptor-positive breast cancer.

Advanced Breast Cancer

Locally advanced breast cancers are treated with chemotherapy before proceeding for surgery. Pre-treatment improves the rate of breast conservation without compromising survival outcomes. Following surgery, all breast-conserving lumpectomies and selected mastectomies should receive radiotherapy to maximize control.

This is followed by chemotherapy for higher response rates in a faster time frame. Selected cases with hormone-positive disease are administered endocrine therapy to suppress the effect of hormones.

Breast Cancer and MHT

The degree of association between breast cancer and MHT remains a controversial issue, particularly in women over fifty. The increased risk of breast cancer with MHT is now believed to be associated with the addition of a synthetic progestogen to estrogen therapy and is related to the duration of use.

The possible increased risk of breast cancer associated with MHT is small and estimated at less than 0.1 per cent per year. It decreases progressively after treatment is stopped. It is similar to or lower than the increased risks associated with common lifestyle factors such as reduced physical activity, obesity and alcohol consumption.

Tibolone, a synthetic steroid with activity on estrogen receptors, does not appear to be associated with any adverse effect on mammographic density, although the risk of breast cancer with tibolone is yet to be fully evaluated in women at low risk of cancer. Micronized progesterone or dydrogesterone is associated with a lower risk of breast cancer than synthetic progestogen.

As a safety measure, annual mammograms should be proposed in case of high breast density in women using MHT.

Management of Cervical Cancer

Cervical cancer is a disease continuum, giving us opportunities over years to treat it in the pre-cancerous phase with complete success. Early diagnosis of early-stage cervical cancers has a good prognosis, with a survival rate of over 90 per cent. In later stages, when pelvic lymph nodes are involved, outcomes are not so good, with survival in less than 60 per cent.

Cervical Intraepithelial Neoplasia (CIN)

Cervical cancer is preceded by CIN, which is a pre-malignant lesion of the cervix that can be diagnosed by Pap smear, colposcopy and cervical biopsy. It develops gradually over the years and provides a window of opportunity for treatment that can prevent cervical cancer.

The management approaches to CIN are:

- Observation with HPV testing, cervical cytology by Pap smear and colposcopy, primarily with CIN 1 and 2.

- Targeted destruction of the lesion or an area on the outside of the cervix called the transformation zone recommended for the higher-grade CIN 3. This is done by excision using cautery in a procedure called LEEP or destruction by cauterization, freezing by cryosurgery or laser treatment.
- Hysterectomy is an option for the higher grades of CIN in the perimenopause to avoid the need for regular and long-term follow up.

Early-Stage Cervical Cancer

Since the tumour is largely limited to the cervix, early-stage cervical cancer offers an opportunity for definitive treatment.

Early-stage cervical cancers are treated initially with surgery:

- Conization, which excises the entire disease with clear margins conserving the cervix and the uterus.
- Simple hysterectomy for patients who desire definitive treatment and have completed childbearing is favoured in the perimenopause.
- Modified radical hysterectomy where the uterus, cervix, upper part of the vagina and the tissues around the uterus are removed.
- Lymphadenectomy where the lymph nodes in the pelvis are removed to stage the disease.

Surgery may be followed by radiation therapy and chemotherapy:

- Radiation is highly effective in most cervical cancers and may be given externally and/or internally through the vagina.
- Chemotherapy is used for high-risk disease that is beyond the surgical margin or where the lymph nodes are involved.

Advanced Cervical Cancer

Locally advanced cervical cancer is when the disease has invaded beyond the uterus reaching the pelvic sidewall or involves the rectum or bladder.

Locally advanced cervical cancer is treated with primary chemotherapy rather than primary surgery followed by:

- Radical hysterectomy where the uterus, cervix, upper part of the vagina and the tissues around the uterus are removed with a lymphadenectomy where the lymph nodes in the pelvis are removed to stage the disease.
- Extended field radiation therapy.

Cervical Cancer and MHT

For patients with cervical cancer with menopausal symptoms following treatment, MHT is a safe treatment option since this cancer is not affected by hormones.

Management of Uterine Cancer

Post-menopausal bleeding (PMB) is defined as uterine bleeding occurring after at least one year of menopause. PMB should be considered as caused by uterine (endometrial) cancer until proven otherwise, although only 1–14 per cent of such patients will actually have cancer. After menopause, an endometrial thickness over 5 mm needs investigation so that suspicious lesions in the uterus can be diagnosed early.

Of course, a more common cause of PMB is a thinned-out, atrophic endometrium, so be assured that not all bleeding at this time is because of cancer.

Medical or surgical management of high-risk, endometrial hyperplasia has the potential of preventing uterine cancer. Early-stage, low-risk, uterine cancers have good prognosis with a survival rate of over 95 per cent. Outcomes are worse once pelvic lymph nodes are involved, with survival in 70 per cent.

Endometrial Hyperplasia

Endometrial hyperplasia is an overgrowth of the lining of the uterus and is categorized into two types, based on which management is decided:

• Hyperplasia without atypia (abnormality of cells that could be pre-cancerous).

• Hyperplasia with atypia which can progress to endometrial carcinoma.

The diagnosis of endometrial hyperplasia and the type is made by aspiration cytology, D and C and hysteroscopy where the cavity of the uterus is examined using a telescope called a hysteroscope.

The choice of treatment is based on the presence or absence of atypia, menopausal status and other risk factors:

- Observation is a reasonable alternative before menopause when there are no risk factors for endometrial carcinoma.
- Progestin therapy using oral progesterone, COCs or levonorgestrel-releasing intrauterine device (Mirena) reduces the risk of progression to endometrial cancer.
- Hysterectomy is recommended for hyperplasia with atypia after menopause and if childbearing is complete before menopause.

Early-Stage Uterine Cancer

Low-risk disease is diagnosed if the tumour has the following characteristics:

- Low grade on histology.
- Cancer limited to the endometrium or invading less than one-half of the uterine muscle.
- Cancer that is not a high-risk type such as clear cell, serous, or carcinosarcoma.

The treatment is primarily surgical and includes:

- Total hysterectomy, removal of both tubes and ovaries and evaluation of the lymph nodes.
- Followed by surveillance only rather than any additional therapy.

Advanced Uterine Cancer

While the majority of uterine cancers are localized with an excellent prognosis, a small number present with metastasis. For these, the treatment is more palliative than curative.

The treatment involves multiple modalities:

- Cytoreduction to remove as much of the cancer as possible for newly diagnosed metastatic disease.
- Chemotherapy.
- Endocrine therapy with HER 2-positive cancers.
- Immune therapy for progression despite prior chemotherapy.

Uterine Cancer and MHT

Unopposed estrogen therapy is associated with a duration and dose-related increase in risk of endometrial hyperplasia and uterine cancer. However, the simple addition of a progestogen has again been shown to reduce the risk of uterine cancer associated with estrogen therapy and should always be used except in women who have undergone hysterectomy.

Progestogen treatment could be with oral medication or the levonorgestrel-releasing intrauterine system (Mirena).

Tibolone, which is also used as a form of MHT, does not induce endometrial hyperplasia or uterine cancer in post-menopausal women.

The long-term use of tamoxifen after the treatment of breast cancer has a small but definite association with endometrial hyperplasia and uterine cancer. Women on this treatment should have the endometrial thickness checked regularly.

Management of Ovarian Cancer

Ovarian cancer is predominantly a disease of post-menopausal women with an increase in prevalence with an increasingly aged population. Over 95 per cent of ovarian cancers arise from the surface epithelium of the ovary with the remaining arising from other ovarian cells such as germ cells and the stromal cells in the ovarian substance.

By virtue of the ovaries being difficult to access and because spread of cancer is rapid because the ovaries are in the abdomen, many women experience symptoms only in the later stages of disease leading to them presenting late for treatment. While early-stage, low-risk uterine cancers have a relatively good prognosis with survival rate of over 90 per cent, outcomes are worse with spread in the abdomen with survival in just 40 per cent.

Early-Stage Ovarian Cancer

In early-stage disease, the tumour is still within one or both ovaries.

The treatment is a combination of surgical and medical treatment:

- Total hysterectomy, removal of both tubes and ovaries, removal of the lymph nodes and the omentum, which is a curtain of fat within the abdomen.
- Chemotherapy.

Advanced Ovarian Cancer

A majority of ovarian cancers present in later stages with local or distant metastasis (spread). For these, the treatment is palliative rather than curative.

The treatment involves multiple modalities:

- Cytoreduction to remove as much of the cancer as possible for newly diagnosed metastatic disease.
- Chemotherapy.

For women who are not candidates for surgery or medical therapy and those who have recurrent disease, treatment is palliative, not curative, with the goal of keeping them comfortable.

Pre-existing Cancers and MHT

MHT is neutral and can be used with cervical cancer, most types of ovarian cancer, endometrial cancer (adenocarcinoma), haematological cancers, skin cancers, colorectal cancer, liver cancer, prolactinoma, kidney cancer, pancreatic cancer and thyroid cancer.

MHT is contraindicated and should not be used with breast cancer, endometrial cancer (sarcoma), uterine carcinosarcoma, estrogen dependent ovarian cancer and hormone receptor-positive gastric and bladder cancer.

If systemic, MHT is not recommended, low-dose, local, vaginal estrogen therapy may be used for the treatment of vaginal dryness related to hormone deficiency after most types of cancer.

13

Fertility, Reproduction and Contraception

'And you begin again and sometimes you lose, sometimes you win, but you begin again. Even though your heart is breaking, in time the sun will shine and you will begin again.'

—Barry Manilow

I love stories so here is mine yet again. I entered my adult years dead sure I was going to have children at some point in my life. I had named my three kids by the age of twenty-one, was subscribed to a parenting magazine and read everything there was on parenting at the time. I got married at twenty-six but things didn't quite work out though that's not the story here. Given my situation, I consciously made a decision not to plan kids. After I got divorced, I got busy studying again and landing back on my feet. I have always told Dr Nozer that I wanted kids, but coming from a solid, two-parent home, I didn't want to raise a child by myself. As my friend, Dilshad, says, maybe I made excuses; if I had really wanted kids, I would have had them. But I was looking for a solid relationship which did not happen for me. Believe me when I say this, the acceptance that I could not have kids was a 'painful' experience for me, very painful. In retrospect, I should have, maybe, just gone ahead. I had many conversations with Dr Nozer, he told me my test results were great and I could go ahead at any time, a friend volunteered to be the sperm donor, I searched sperm banks, froze my eggs and I still did not do it. My advice to my younger self at that time would be: 'Do it!'

Shonali Sabherwal

R came to me last year when she was fifty years old and married for four years. She was keen to conceive. Her FSH levels were 14 and her AMH, which is a mark of her ovarian reserve, less than 0.03. These levels suggested that she was well into perimenopause. She was made to understand the medical risks of having a pregnancy at this age and first underwent an assessment of medical fitness to carry a pregnancy herself. On her request, we did a cycle of ovulation induction, to which there was no ovarian response. We counselled her about the option of undergoing an IVF using eggs from a suitable donor, which she did. Her first cycle of IVF was a success, and she had a twin pregnancy. We did have our challenges with hypertension and a few other medical issues, but she had a relatively seamless pregnancy. She was fifty-one years and six months old when she delivered a healthy baby girl and a healthy baby boy by caesarean section a month before her due date. R and her husband are a simple couple who married late in life. They decided to go ahead with their dream family, and it was a privilege for us to have used advanced technology and good old obstetric care to have made their dream a reality.

Nozer Sheriar

A woman's ability to get pregnant begins to decrease slightly starting at the age of twenty-seven years and significantly reduces by the age of thirty-seven. That is not to say that age is an absolute barrier, since many women are having babies in their mid- and late-thirties and even in their early- or mid-forties. Some have a spontaneous pregnancy; others need medical assistance, which could be basic or advanced. Technically, with the availability of assisted reproductive technologies (ART) and the use of donor eggs, menopause is no longer the final frontier or a barrier to motherhood.

How Does One Plan a Pregnancy in Midlife?

If you know in your heart that you'd like to become a parent then, in this day and age, you should just go ahead. There are many options that did not exist before. My cousin, who was exactly like me, but in a super-loving relationship, finally had her baby after twenty-one years of married life through surrogacy with her eggs at the age of forty-six. So yes, it can be done.

I am healthy and I had this preconceived notion that I could conceive at any age, but my ovaries are not concerned with whether I am Macrobiotic, sugar-free or dairy-free. There are a fixed number of eggs you have in a lifespan and this number and quality decreases with age. This ageing of the ovaries is hard to escape. So, then you have to look for options. There are fertility treatments, IVF considerations, surrogacy with a donor egg and in case you are single, using donor sperm. It's a challenge that you have to be up for. But I say it again: 'just do it!'

Shonali Sabherwal

If after the age of thirty, a woman does not conceive naturally within six months of trying for pregnancy, the couple should have a fertility workup. She should undergo ovarian reserve testing by measuring AMH levels, although these are known to vary widely. Many women do spontaneously conceive even with very low levels of AMH, so you should never be disheartened. There is a role for using dehydroepiandrosterone (DHEAS) to improve ovarian function in such cases.

In women aged over forty, who do not conceive within two to four cycles of standard fertility treatment, where ovulation is tracked and relations are timed, IUI and then IVF should be considered.

The only effective fertility treatment for ovarian ageing, close to or after menopause, when ovaries significantly reduce or cease to function, is oocyte donation since pregnancy rates associated with this treatment are significantly higher than those associated with controlled ovarian stimulation or IVF with the woman's own eggs.

Preconception counselling, work up and preparation is vital when planning a pregnancy in midlife, with an emphasis on optimal general health and screening for medical conditions, such as hypertension, diabetes, and pregnancy-related risks. A pregnancy in a healthy older woman may actually be safer than that in an unhealthy, out-of-shape, younger woman.

How Safe are Pregnancies in the Midlife?

It goes to reason that as age increases, women run a higher risk of pregnancy issues and complications. Miscarriage rates are higher, risk of genetic abnormalities (particularly trisomy 21, the technical name for Down's syndrome, where there is an extra chromosome 21 causing mental retardation) are significantly increased, congenital birth defects in the foetus are more frequent and medical disorders such as preeclampsia (hypertension in pregnancy) and gestational diabetes are more common.

It can be more challenging to maintain your health while pregnant the closer you are to fifty. According to Mary Jane

Minkin, Clinical Professor of Obstetrics and Gynaecology at Yale University the risks of becoming hypersensitive and diabetic increase with age and become magnified with pregnancy. besides during pregnancy, the heart has to work 50 per cent harder than in the non-pregnant state and the circulating fluid volume goes up by a full 50 per cent creating an additional risk of heart disease.

Of course, a big part of the outcomes depends on how healthy the women going into pregnancies are. Many women do well and with vigilance and pre-natal testing, achieve near-normal outcomes.

The pre-natal tests would include:

- Ultrasounds, which will be used to rule out birth defects and to monitor the growth and wellbeing of your baby.
- Blood tests indicating how you are doing on various parameters.
- Chorionic villus sampling (CVS), sampling baby's tissues.
- Amniocentesis, to sample your amniotic fluid.
- Non-invasive pre-natal tests (NIPT) to check chromosomes by assessing cell-free foetal DNA.

Is It Safe and Advisable to Be an Elderly Mother?

One argument on the benefits of having children later in life points to the fact that older parents live longer. Later pregnancies also protect against cognitive decline, which means you stay sharper in the brain. A diverse group of women was studied by the University of Southern California between the ages of forty-one and ninety-two. Their research, published in the *Journal of the American Geriatrics Society*, provides strong evidence of a

> . . . positive association between later age at last pregnancy
> and late-life cognition and mental health.[*]

Also, if you are older, chances are you are better settled in a career, less worried about survival stuff like job security and therefore, more focused on your kids and their upbringing. In an article that appeared on the nytimes.com portal on 'Good News for Older Moms', the researcher Tea Trillingsgaard says,

> Older mothers have more psychological flexibility, more cognitive flexibility, more ability to tolerate complex emotional stimuli from the children.[†]

Do You Need to Continue Contraception in the Perimenopause?

Women in perimenopause do have lower fertility but pregnancies are possible at any age until ovarian function packs up for good. In fact, couples at this phase in their lives tend to let down their guard because they don't expect to get pregnant, so unwanted pregnancies do occur. Many women may even fail to diagnose the pregnancy for the longest time since they may already have irregular or delayed periods or assume menopause has arrived. This may increase the need for late abortion to manage pregnancies that need termination.

---

[*] 'Women Who Have Their Last Baby after 35 Are Mentally Sharper in Old Age, Study Finds', *Journal of the American Geriatrics Society*.
[†] Trillingsgaard, Tea, 'Good News for Older Moms', *New York Times*, 3 April 2017.

With this background, the importance of contraception in the perimenopause cannot be stressed enough. An entire basket of contraceptive choices, both temporary and permanent, is available and the selection depends on a woman's situation, her health and her preferences.

Sterilization by tubal ligation is a highly effective, safe, single act and is a permanent method. Vasectomy for the male partner is considered even safer. The use of long-acting, reversable contraception (LARC), such as intrauterine devices, injectables and implants, has marginalized permanent surgical methods to a great extent. Although intrauterine-contraceptive devices are effective, medicated copper devices sometimes can cause heavy and painful periods.

Oral contraceptive pills (OCPs) are effective, easy to use, and reversible. Low-dose OCPs have many non-contraceptive health benefits with an increased safety profile. For women above the age of thirty-five, using OCPs, a careful assessment of personal and family history and accurate measurement of blood pressure (BP), breast examination, screening for diabetes and lipid profile should be performed. Healthy women of normal weight, non-users of tobacco and those doing well on a combination contraceptive pill can continue this method until the age of menopause and up to a year or two years later, after analysing its risks and benefits. Change over from contraceptive pills to MHT is carried out between an arbitrary age of forty-five and fifty years, if serum FSH is over 30 IU/L.

The long-acting injectable, contraceptive depot medroxyprogesterone acetate (DMPA) is associated with bone loss, which returns to normal, after stopping DMPA. Yet caution needs to be exercised in women at high risk of osteoporosis.

Progesterone-only contraceptive is an ideal method in women with a history of venous thromboembolism (VTE) and gallstones. Its limitations are the resultant erratic and scanty periods. The levonorgestrel-intrauterine system (Mirena), apart from being used as a contraceptive, is an effective therapy for heavy menstrual bleeding and for treating bleeding disturbances associated with endometrial hyperplasia.

Emergency contraception is an effective emergency method, particularly when sex is infrequent during perimenopause, but it is not as effective and consistent as the use of other contraceptives.

Snapshot on Lifestyle and Diet

Lifestyle Recommendations

- All inversions in yoga will help with fertility (the exercise section has detailed poses listed), as also pelvic-floor exercises including core work.
- Stay in control of your weight; obesity does not help, so exercise is key.
- Get rid of chemicals in your environment. Exposure to endocrine disruptors (EDCs) plays havoc with your hormones, reduces the quality of sperm and eggs and affect the chances of your getting pregnant.
- Avoid air fresheners, heavily perfumed products and plastic fumes, smells and paint since they all contain EDCs.
- Drink water from a glass bottle.
- Quit smoking.

- Avoid heavy use of antibiotics unless necessary.
- Pay attention to the kind of lubricant beings used while having sex as some of them affect conception.
- Minimize alcohol.
- Pay attention to your oral health. Infections and inflammation in the mouth have been linked to increased risk of developing pre-eclampsia, premature birth and having a baby with lower birth weight.

Diet Recommendations

- Stay away from sugar, dairy, refined, processed and packaged foods.
- Keep coffee (caffeine) under moderation.
- Change your salt to sea, rock or Himalayan pink salt.
- Avoid trans fats in commercial foods.
- Change to cold-pressed oils since they do not cause free radical damage.
- Nuts, avocados, olive oil and grapeseed oil can help reducing inflammation, which promotes fertility and ovulation.
- Make sure you eat foods that are home cooked and focus on whole grains (complex carbohydrates such as millet, brown rice and barley are fertility-friendly and full of vitamins B and E, including many antioxidants).
- Buckwheat has the compound d-chiro-inositol, which improves ovulation.
- Try staying more plant-based.
- Those with PCOS can avoid gluten altogether as it creates an inflammatory response and that may not help fertility. Include lean protein—fish and chicken—and good sources of zinc, iron all important for a healthy

pregnancy. Vegetarians stick to both kinds of beans, the whole and split (lentils). Processed soy should be avoided; tofu is okay to include.

- Have 2–3 juices made from greens (between meals), with carrot and avocado for good fats. Rotate greens by using different greens every week.
- Add spirulina.
- Use fermented foods to keep the gut healthy (see the diet section).

Medical Treatment for Infertility in Midlife

Reproductive-age women should be aware that natural fertility and ART success, except with egg donation, is significantly lower for women in their late thirties and forties.

Fertility Enhancement and Treatment in Midlife

There is no doubt that fertility in midlife decreases year after year until, in women forty years and older, fertility is significantly less than when they were younger. This fertility potential is reflected in their AMH levels. Because of the decline in fertility that leads to an increased time to conception that occurs after the age of thirty-five years, women at this age should be referred for infertility work-up after six months of trying to conceive naturally.

There are women who reach menopause later than others, who continue to ovulate normally and who continue to have fertility better than average. Yet others may need medical assistance in the form of ovarian stimulation by medication which may be combined with intrauterine insemination

(IUI). Finally, for women over forty years of age, who wish to use their own eggs, assisted reproduction (ART) offers the best chances for conception and delivery. The only effective treatment for ovarian ageing is oocyte donation and a woman with significantly decreased ovarian reserve should be offered oocyte donation as an option, as pregnancy rates associated with this treatment are significantly higher.

Women planning conception late in life for whatever reason have the following options.

Planned Relations

Timing sex by using the calendar method, urine ovulation test kits or ultrasound-follicular study, either in unstimulated natural cycles or in ovulation-induction cycles with oral clomiphene citrate or letrozole. Since pregnancy rates are extremely low in comparison with younger women, least amount of time should be spent on planned relations and the more advanced treatments should be sought early.

Intrauterine Insemination (IUI)

Undertaken in natural or ovulation-induction cycles with oral clomiphene citrate or letrozole or injections of gonadotropins, IUI is guided by an ultrasound follicular study. Since pregnancy rates are below 5 per cent, IUI may be undertaken in two to three cycles before opting for ART.

Assisted Reproductive Technologies (ART)

In vitro fertilization (IVF) and intracytoplasmic sperm injection (ICSI) are undertaken either with the woman's own eggs or eggs from a younger, more fertile, donor. In women over forty, the live birth rate for each ART cycle is around 15 per cent with their own eggs and over 30 per cent with donor eggs. These are the highest success rates treatment can achieve and IVF must be offered as an option early in the treatment.

Surrogacy

This is an option for women with major health issues that make carrying a pregnancy to term dangerous or where the uterus is not capable of supporting or retaining a pregnancy. Here, another woman, younger and in good health, carries the pregnancy for the woman, using the couple's embryos.

Pregnancies in Midlife

The average age of pregnancy, both the first and subsequent, has steadily increased. In our practice, we have well over a hundred over-forty pregnancies, with a mean age of 42.1 years, with 40 per cent having their first pregnancy. A third conceived naturally, a third with fertility treatment including IUI and a third with ART.

While elderly women are believed to experience many risks associated with pregnancy, with adequate planning and preparation, they do quite well obstetrically. In fact, most women planning a pregnancy in midlife have maintained good physical health, often better than younger counterparts. So, age is no longer a reason not to try if a baby is wanted.

Nozer Sheriar

Preparing for Pregnancy

The preparation for pregnancy includes counselling regarding the risks of pregnancy with advanced maternal age, promotion of optimal health and weight and screening and treatment of medical conditions such as hypertension and diabetes. Incidentally, advanced paternal age also appears to be associated with an increased risk of miscarriage, genetic conditions and autism spectrum disorders.

Miscarriages

While miscarriage risk is believed to be about 15 per cent across all pregnancies, it doubles after the age of forty because of chromosomal problems in the embryo. Because of older eggs, women are likely to have a miscarriage in over one in three elderly pregnancies. To mitigate the risk, the early stages of late-in-life pregnancies are given additional support with progesterone medication.

Congenital Anomalies

Once again, the older an egg, the more likely it is to have chromosomal abnormalities, which can increase the child's risk for certain birth defects. Trisomy 21 (Down syndrome), associated with mental retardation and other typical features, is the most common chromosomal condition in women who get pregnant at an older age. At the age of twenty-five, the risk of trisomy 21 is one in 1500, with the risk jumping to one in 100 at the age of forty years. Every woman is recommended routine genetic testing by NIPT (non-invasive pre-natal testing), chorion villus sampling or amniocentesis during early or mid-pregnancy with the option of medical termination if an abnormality is detected.

Medical Disorders

With age, the chances of developing cardiovascular problems like high blood pressure and heart disease increase. Pregnant women over forty are at higher risk for pre-eclampsia (high blood pressure during pregnancy which can be life threatening), diabetes in pregnancy and thyroid disease. These conditions can create problems for both mother and baby, including low or abnormally high birth weights and premature deliveries. The involvement of other specialists such as cardiologists and endocrinologists helps make such pregnancies safer.

Other problems are a higher incidence of fibroids with pregnancy and placenta previa, a condition in which the placenta either partly or fully covers the cervix. Both can increase the risk for premature birth and excess bleeding after delivery.

Preventing Stillbirths

Pregnant women in their forties are at higher risk of stillbirth because of conditions like high blood pressure or diabetes during pregnancy. These pregnancies are considered high risk and need intense vigilance with frequent follow up, ultrasound and foetal monitoring. Also, because longer gestational times can increase the risk of stillbirth, a woman over forty is preferably delivered before her due date.

Safe Modes of Delivery

It is a common assumption that the elderly woman must be delivered by a caesarean section, which is not true. Over a third of the over-forty pregnancies in our practice deliver normally, with it being the preferred option. The labour is monitored closely and pain relief is provided with an epidural. Given this, it is important to discuss safe-delivery options and respect a woman's choice.

14

Premature Ovarian Failure or Insufficiency

'Aging gracefully is one thing, but trying to slow it down is another.'

—Courteney Cox

My friend always wanted kids. I knew she would be a super mom. I saw this in the way she interacted with children; her need to nurture was always a strong point. When she conceived, I thought to myself, this is it. Sadly, she lost the baby at five months, when she had to terminate the pregnancy because of some complications. She lives in New York, so we meet once a year. I met her a year after she had lost her baby, when she asked me to accompany her to go see an alternative medical practitioner, someone who would give her some herbs to calm down. She has always been an anxious personality, but after losing the baby, it had really gone bad for her. She tried to get pregnant again but met with no luck and the next year I met her she had gone through her menopause. She was only forty at the time. I have seen many women who go through early menopause and the reasons for this are multifold. However, it does not mean women can't have children, enjoy a sexual relationship or look great after forty.

Shonali Sabherwal

S came to me when she was twenty-seven years old, never having had a period on her own without hormonal medication. She now had regular light periods by being on a contraceptive pill. Her FSH levels were 72 and estradiol levels less than 20, leading us to a diagnosis of premature ovarian failure or ovarian insufficiency. The ultrasound revealed an underdeveloped uterus with a thin endometrial lining; DEXA scan diagnosed osteopenia and her genetic tests revealed the normal female genetic pattern of 46XX with two X chromosomes. I started her on estrogen therapy and over six months, the uterine size increased to near normal dimensions. To this, we then added progesterone with which she started with her regular normal periods. This was supplemented with calcium and weight-bearing exercise for bone health. A big part of our care was confidence building, counselling regarding her condition and relationship guidance, where I stressed honesty and transparency. Then, one day she met with her soulmate online with whom she shared information about her premature ovarian insufficiency. She even brought her potential mother-in-law to meet me and we spoke about her condition and laid out her fertility options. She is now happily married and living overseas. She is on MHT and has planned for pregnancy with egg donation after two years. Of course, the MHT will continue for at least another twenty years, until the expected age of menopause. I have nothing but the greatest admiration for S, her honesty and her belief in herself. Others would be shamed by the stigma and choose to hide their condition, but not she. Thankfully, medical advances have made pregnancy a reality for women for whom it was earlier an impossibility.

Nozer Sheriar

When Is Menopause Considered Premature?

Menopause occurring before the age of forty is known as premature ovarian failure, premature menopause or premature ovarian insufficiency (POI). It can occur naturally or as a result of medical or surgical treatment. It is characterized by typical menopausal symptoms and signs, including delayed or absent periods and elevated FSH levels. Conventionally, the diagnosis of frank POI is made if there are no periods for three to four months and FSH levels over 40 IU/L are repeated a month apart. Recent European

Society of Human Reproduction and Embryology (ESHRE) guidelines diagnose POI if there are delayed or no periods for at least four months and the FSH level is over 25 IU/L.

The incidence of spontaneous POI is 1 per cent of women under the age of forty and 0.1 per cent of women under the age of thirty. The incidence of iatrogenic POI (caused by surgery and medical treatments) may be growing due to increasing survival rates following chemotherapy and radiotherapy for various cancers, which leave survivors with poor or absent ovarian function.

Women with POI are now recognized to be at increased risk for premature health issues and mortality. They have a higher risk of ischemic heart disease, stroke, fractures due to osteoporosis and diminished sexual wellbeing.

How Is Premature Ovarian Insufficiency Diagnosed?

POI may be either primary, where menstruation has never occurred, or secondary, where menstruation ceases after previous spontaneous periods. In the majority of cases of primary POI, the cause is genetic, with abnormalities such as Turner syndrome (single X chromosome), mosaicism and deletions and rearrangements of the X chromosome. Secondary POI may be caused by removal of or damage to the ovaries by surgery, disease, radiation or chemotherapy.

Diagnosis is based on the following:

- Information on menopausal symptoms such as hot flushes, vaginal dryness, lack of libido, bone and joint pains, loss of concentration, insomnia and fertility issues.
- History of previous medical or surgical treatment.
- Family history of POI.

- No or infrequent periods, taking into account whether the woman has a uterus.
- Vaginal examination.
- Ultrasound scanning.
- Hormone analysis with high FSH levels at least 4–6 weeks apart. AMH testing is not to be used for the diagnosis.
- Thyroid and adrenal antibody assays.
- Karyotyping and detection of fragile X syndrome.

Snapshot on Lifestyle and Diet

A lot of what women go through post-menopause is what women go through in premature ovarian insufficiency as well. While the diet and exercise sections outline everything in great detail, here is a snapshot of what women should do.

During this time the adrenal system is put under tremendous pressure due to the peaks and lows of hormonal fluctuations. Any additional stressors on a food-and-choice-of-beverages front, will increase the strain on the adrenals and trigger as well as worsen many menopause-like symptoms you are already going through. The muscles and bones will need attention since the decline in estrogen turns some of our muscles to fat and also leaches out calcium from our bones. We need our muscles to support the skeletal system and avoid any injuries. We must strive for flexibility in our joints. Getting a frozen shoulder, hip and lower back pain are very common during this time.

Lifestyle Recommendations

- Yoga can help women of all ages and all stages of menopause, especially women with premature ovarian insufficiency (POI). A regular practice of gentle stretching and strengthening, with breathing and meditation exercises that calm the nervous system and bring a sense of mental clarity and equilibrium helps. Yoga has long-term physical and emotional benefits, so including it daily is important. If you are a beginner, then start with a Hatha yoga class, slowly building up your practice to Ashtanga or Iyengar style of yoga, whatever works.

- Stay on top of your weight; obesity does not help, so exercise is key.
- Journaling always helps to stay on top of what you are going through and analyse how you are feeling. It also provides an escape mechanism for any bottled-up emotions that may stress you out further.
- Try psychotherapy if you get extremely stressed out.
- Drink water from a glass or copper bottle.
- Quit smoking.
- Join a women's group or get into a team activity. You may join a laughter group or link up with women who meet on a regular basis to go out and lighten up.
- Use extra lubrication while having sex.
- If you were hoping to get pregnant and have not, then be open to talk to your partner about it. Share your feelings about what you may be going through, viz-à-viz not having a child. You may want to explore more options on other ways of having a child—through adoption or surrogacy
- Give yourself time to accept your diagnosis; it is always a gradual process of acceptance. Focus on the good things like your diet.

Diet Recommendations

While all the recommendations are important in the diet section, here is a snapshot of what you can stay focused on.

- Stay away from the following foods: sugar, dairy (minimize if you can't eliminate), processed or packaged or refined foods. These will only cause a further deterioration of the blood condition, causing it to get acidic, throw off the pH balance and also destroy gut bacteria, further complicating the impact on bones, joints, tissues and lead to a toxin build-up.
- Minimize alcohol, as this will stress the adrenal glands.
- Avoid heavy use of antibiotics or anti-depressants unless necessary. These will impact the ecosystem of your gut, diminishing good gut bacteria.
- Keep coffee (caffeine) under moderation; it does not help adrenal glands.
- Change your salt to sea, rock or Himalayan pink salt.
- Avoid trans fats (commercial foods). Change to cold-pressed oils—they do not cause free radical damage. Focus on healthy fats—nuts, avocados, olive oil and grapeseed oil can also help reduce inflammation.
- Make sure you eat foods that are home-cooked and focus on whole grains like millet, brown rice and barley which are full of B and E vitamins and include many antioxidants. Buckwheat can be a great gluten-free option at this time as gluten creates an inflammatory response.
- Focus on lentil, beans, good quality lean protein like fish and chicken which are good sources of zinc and iron, all important for immunity. Chia and flax seeds

have essential fatty acids and grapes, berries, plums, green and black tea have antioxidants. Processed soy should be avoided but tofu is okay to include.

- Have 2–3 greens juices a day in-between meals with a carrot and avocado for good fats, using different greens every week.
- Add spirulina (sea vegetable).
- Use fermented foods to keep the gut healthy.
- Add curcumin (capsules are okay) to keep the inflammatory response of the body in check.
- Add collagen in the form of powder or a bone broth.

Medical Management of Premature Ovarian Insufficiency

It is important to inform the woman of this difficult diagnosis with empathy, in a sensitive and caring manner. Women must be provided with adequate information and counselling about POI, consequences and solutions.

MHT for Premature Ovarian Insufficiency

All women with POI should receive MHT after excluding contraindications. Appropriate counselling, lifestyle modification and MHT with estrogen, progesterone and possibly testosterone form the mainstay of treatment. MHT should be started as early as possible in women with POI and continued until the average age of natural menopause. There is no evidence that MHT for POI increases risk of breast cancer, CVD or dementia, over and above that found in menstruating women with a normally timed menopause.

Higher doses of estrogens compared to women over forty years are usually required. The recommended estrogen doses are estradiol 2 mg/day or 1.25mg conjugated equine estrogen (CEE) or transdermal estradiol 75–100 mg/day or 10 ug ethinyl estradiol. The aim is to achieve the typical mean serum estradiol levels of approximately 100 pg/ml, found in regularly menstruating women. Micronized progesterone can be administered as a cyclic regimen (200 mg for 12 days each month) or as a continuous regimen of 100 mg per day.

In women with low libido, especially where ovaries have been surgically removed, testosterone gels or patches could be used along with MHT on a case-by-case basis.

The risk of diseases such as breast cancer and cardiovascular disease increases with age and is very low in women aged under forty years. Both MHT and combined oral contraceptives offer bone protection. MHT may have a beneficial effect on blood pressure as compared to a combined oral contraceptive.

Combined estrogen/progestogen contraceptive pills (COCs) may also be used continuously until the expected time of the menopause. MHT is not contraceptive unless estrogen is combined with a levonorgestrel intrauterine system. It may therefore be more practical for the COC to be used for the first few years following diagnosis of POI in those wishing to avoid pregnancy.

Supplementary Therapy for Premature Ovarian Insufficiency

Osteopenia and osteoporosis are a major concern with POI. Prevention with heathy lifestyle, weight-bearing-bone-strengthening exercises and calcium and vitamin D supplementation should be started early.

Regular assessment of bone density with early treatment with bisphosphonates for osteopenia or strontium ranelate or denosumab for osteoporosis.

Pregnancies in Premature Ovarian Insufficiency

IVF with donor oocyte is a successful treatment choice for women with POI.

- The preparation for pregnancy starts well before with extended estrogen treatment to develop a uterus of adequate size and shape to carry a pregnancy.
- The donor undergoes ovarian stimulation and the embryo, fresh or frozen, is transferred into the uterus with a well-prepared endometrium.
- The endometrium is first prepared with estradiol and the pregnancy post-transfer supported by estrogen and progesterone through the duration of the first trimester.
- This may be supplemented pre-transfer with sildenafil and low dose aspirin thereafter.
- By 12 weeks, the placenta is formed and takes on the entire hormonal function of supporting the pregnancy. Then medical support becomes unnecessary.

There is also the option of transplantation of fresh ovarian tissue or ovarian transplantation, with many successful pregnancies reported. Transplantation carries with it the risk of major surgery and long-term immunosuppressant therapy, and this should be part of counselling, particularly since the safer option of donor oocytes is available.

Modern medicine has ensured the option of pregnancy in women with POI if they so desire and this must be conveyed to them early on.

15

Menopause Hormone Therapy: To Do or Not to Do?

'It's supposed to be a secret, but I'll tell you anyway. We doctors do nothing. We only help. And encourage the doctor within.'

—Albert Schweitzer

Poonam, my friend, went through a really hard time with her pre-menopausal state; she called me one day to say she was terribly depressed, found it difficult to get out of bed, had gained weight.

She said to me, 'I am going to die.'

It is at times like this that I feel bad I have friends who live out of the country, because I wish I could just run over and be with them. So, since I could not, as she lives in Canada, I tried my very best to support her through phone calls. But it just wasn't working. We lost touch for a while, you know how the business of life can take over, but she remained in my prayers every day.

A couple of months later, she called and said, 'Honey I am fine and feel amazing, all thanks to HRT.' She said it had saved her and this ran so contrary to what my views were (through my research and understanding) on HRT. This is when my mindset changed on the subject.

Shonali Sabherwal

R, an actor, a lovely mother of two, first consulted me when she was thirty-two years old. A known case of PCOS with concerns about her skin, which was prone to acne and rashes, she exercised regularly and was amazingly fit. She did well on oral contraceptive pills, which she continued for most of the next sixteen years. When she stopped the pill, she experienced perimenopausal symptoms for which she was placed on biosimilar hormone therapy with limited benefit. This is when she started showing the most unpredictable hormonal patterns. Initially, her FSH levels were normal, and her estradiol levels elevated to well above 300, probably a consequence of the biosimilar estrogens. For the next year, she was treated with monthly cycles of natural progesterone to balance the estrogen excess and maintain regular periods.

At the end of a year, she experienced symptoms of hot flushes, exhaustion, vaginal dryness, hair loss and breakouts of acne and her FSH levels were in the menopausal range. Now, R is a person totally involved with every decision we make, and she would regularly test hormone levels to try to make sense of what she was going through, even though I did not ask her to do so. Over the next twelve months, the results were confounding: her FSH levels ranged from fifteen to seventy-five and estradiol from seventeen to 330, as if her ovaries were fighting to keep going. We started transdermal estrogen gel in different doses and this worked well to alleviate her symptoms. While the flushes were controlled, moods benefited, vaginal dryness resolved and periods became regular, she began to experience hormonal headaches akin to migraine. She is presently on a hormonal break to allow us to reassess her symptoms with the option of later moving to tibolone. R is an amazing patient to work with. She is involved and engaged and makes me think, often outside the box. She signifies for me the unique needs of every case and the importance of individualizing our approach to the perimenopause.

Nozer Sheriar

Why has HRT historically got a bad rap?

Estrogen-replacement therapy was born in the late 1950s, an era when women thought their lives were over after menopause. Back then, it was believed that women's jobs finished after bearing children, as was their youthfulness. After bearing children, they were of no use to their husbands and not considered sexually attractive as they approached menopause. The advent of ERT, to make them feel better and stay youthful, was viewed as an intervention that kept them 'young forever'. ERT was made popular for mass use in the 1960s. It was not only promoted as palliative, but also promoted as a panacea for women to deal with psychological problems, because of the change in the stage of their lives. Common pre-conceptions made women out to be demons in their pre-menopausal years and projected post-menopausal women as neurotic, asexual, unattractive, leading to the prescription of estrogen without adequate testing.

As a result, from 1965 to the 1970s, ERT became popular and soon became one of the five top-selling prescription drugs. This is when it was reported that cancers in women were growing at an alarming rate, with women on ERT developing uterine (endometrial) cancer at a rate four to eight times greater than in untreated women. The sale of estrogen supplements plummeted and physicians too became reluctant to supply it.

Unopposed estrogen, without the presence of progesterone, was the culprit since cancers were unknown in women whose ovaries produced a proper balance of estrogen and progesterone. When the connection was made to the use of unopposed estrogen, progestins were added to mitigate the effects of estrogen or balance them out and ERT changed to HRT. In women on a combined treatment programme of estrogen and progestin, the incidence of uterine cancer was considerably lower than in women not receiving hormones. The parallel fear of estrogen to be the cause of breast cancer was addressed in the same manner and this brought HRT back to centre stage.

MHT: To Do or Not to Do?

JoAnn Pinkerton, past president of the North American Menopause Society, writes,

> Fear has been driving the conversation about hormone therapy though it remains the most effective treatment for vasomotor symptoms and the genitourinary syndrome of menopause and has been shown to prevent bone loss and fracture.[*]

Hormone therapy is approved by the US FDA for the following indications:

- Vasomotor symptoms such as night sweats, hot flashes and flushes.
- Prevention of bone loss and fractures in post-menopausal women at high risk for osteoporosis or fracture.
- Premature surgical menopause and primary ovarian insufficiency until the average menopausal age is reached.
- Genitourinary menopausal symptoms, where low-dose vaginal estrogen therapy is first-line, rather than systemic therapy.

---

[*] Pinkerton, Jo Ann V., 'Changing the Conversation about Hormone Therapy', *Menopause the Journal of the North American Menopause Society*, Vol. 24 (9), September 2017, pp. 991–93.

Since the 2002 publication of findings from the Women's Health Initiative (WHI), anxiety about risk for breast cancer, heart disease and dementia have dominated clinical discussions about hormone therapy. However, follow-up data from the WHI shows no increase in cardiovascular diseases, cancer or all-cause mortality.

Dr Pinkerton urges,

> . . . clinicians to change the conversation with women. We want them to feel very comfortable that if a woman is having bothersome menopausal symptoms; hot flashes, night sweats or sleep disturbances, hormone therapy is safe and effective, primarily for women who are starting hormone therapy when they are under 60 and within 10 years of menopause, where there are more benefits than risks.[*]

She emphasizes the differences in risk between estrogen therapy and estrogen with progestin. Estrogen-only therapy, for example, appears to have a better safety profile for longer use.

> The pendulum is swinging back in favor of hormone therapy and it helps clear the air in terms of removing fear and confusion about menopause and the appropriateness of considering hormone therapy . . . The hormone therapy benefits versus risks have been so confusing that the majority of women and many of their doctors still don't accept that the risks are much less than the benefits.[†]

---

[*] Ibid., pp. 91–93.
[†] Ibid.

The applications of MHT are now well established and range from short-term treatment to long-term protection. Symptoms such as hot flushes, night sweats, insomnia and symptoms of vaginal atrophy are easily reversed through hormone therapy. MHT also prevents the central distribution of body fat after menopause, maintaining the pre-menopausal relationship between lean body mass and fat mass. Estrogen remains the drug of choice for preventing of osteoporosis.

What Is the Scope and Types of MHT?

MHT covers therapies including estrogens, progestogens, combined therapies, androgens and tibolone.

- ET—Estrogen therapy.
- EPT—Estrogen-progesterone therapy.
- STEAR—Selective-tissue estrogenic-activity regulators such as tibolone.
- SERMs—Selective estrogen-receptor modulators such as raloxifene.
- AT—Androgen therapy.

Three indications for post-menopausal HT, derived from the results of various clinical trials that have constantly withstood the test of time, are the beneficial effects of estrogens on symptom relief, urogenital atrophy and bone. Besides these, hormone therapy is indicated in POI and early menopause.

MHT is of vital medical importance in the care of an increasing number of ageing women who multitask and simultaneously balance professional, personal and domestic commitments. For symptomatic menopausal woman suffering from hot flushes, insomnia, fatigue and irritability, MHT provides certain relief. It is also necessary for relief from urogenital ageing and vulvovaginal changes that predispose the person to recurrent infections. Besides these short-term benefits, MHT now has an established role in prevention of osteoporosis and cardiovascular disease.

Various formulations, combinations, routes and durations of therapy exist for MHT use. Since no single product or regime can be prescribed for all women, an appreciation of these options can expand the therapeutic choices that women and clinicians can choose from.

How Do You Prepare for and Monitor MHT?

The diagnosis of estrogen deficiency is usually established by the relevant history of menopausal symptoms. The onset of hot flushes and night sweats associated with irregular or absent periods in a woman over forty is virtually diagnostic of the perimenopause. Women must take sufficient time to describe their symptoms. A checklist approach can help guide the enquiry. Information about past or present medical and psychological disturbances and previous therapy must also be discussed.

- A physical examination, including breast, abdominal and pelvic examinations, is mandatory.
- A Pap smear to screen for cervical pathology must be collected.
- Mammography is recommended in women over forty years of age and in younger high-risk patients with a family history of breast cancer or a past history of breast disease.

- Ultrasound is performed to check the ovaries and to screen for ovarian cancer. An internal transvaginal USG is used to assess the endometrium. A post-menopausal endometrial thickness greater than 5 mm is strongly associated with a polyp or adenocarcinoma and must be investigated further.
- Although hormone profiles are not necessary to establish a diagnosis of menopause, at least two sets of FSH and LH values are required to support this diagnosis of menopause.

The dose and duration of use of MHT is individualized and a risk-benefit assessment is carried out annually. Follow-up should be at one month, three months, six months and then annually.

Annual follow-ups are essential when on MHT. A full gynaecological assessment is mandatory and a mammogram or the breast ultrasound should be carried out one to three-yearly if the initial mammogram is normal.

How Is MHT Administered?

MHT can be administered by oral and non-oral routes with the choice of therapy depending on age, your symptoms, presence of the uterus and the purpose of therapy. Treatment plans should be made for no more than a year at a time, and the plans should be tailored to a woman's needs. A single dose one-for-all approach to MHT can never do justice.

MHT using only estrogen

For women who have undergone hysterectomy, daily estrogens are given alone. The addition of progestogens is unnecessary since the need for protecting the endometrium does not exist. This does not apply to patients having undergone endometrial ablation since the possibility of some endometrial glands remaining after surgery is strong.

Estrogen-Progestogen MHT

This is the most frequently used regimen for MHT in women with a uterus. Progestogens in an adequate dose and duration are supplemented along with estrogens. The estrogen corrects the vasomotor disturbances, genitourinary atrophy and prevents osteoporosis and cardiovascular disease. The progestogen is added to protect the endometrium from the development of hyperplasia. The risk of cancer is completely prevented by the administration of cyclic progestogens for ten or more days each month.

In the continuous-cyclic regimen, estrogen is used every day with progestogens added cyclically for ten to fourteen days during each month. The progestogen is started on day one or day fifteen each month. This regimen is suitable for women at perimenopause since uterine bleeding occurs in about 80 per cent of women when progestogen is withdrawn, although bleeding can begin one to two days earlier, depending on the type and dose of progestogen used.

In the continuous-combined regimen, fixed doses of estrogen and progestogen are administered every day. It is the preferred treatment after menopause since most women prefer to avoid withdrawal bleeding with MHT. This regimen successfully avoids withdrawal bleeding in a majority of the users. The incidence of breakthrough bleeding with continuous MHT occurs in 15 per cent of the women.

Combined Hormonal Contraception

Combined low-dose hormonal contraception (the pill or the patch) is a valid MHT option for perimenopausal women. Low-dose combined oral contraception, either triphasic formulations or those with newer progestogens (desogestrel or drosperinone), can be used during this transition period to regularize bleeding and offer contraception to the menstruating woman who is not protected by a permanent method. Although anovulatory cycles increase with age, ovulation can continue until menopause, necessitating birth control. COCs may safely be used up to the age of forty-five and even fifty years when risk factors for hormonal contraception are absent. An extended use of up to three months not only reduces frequency of menses but also benefits VMS.

MHT Using Only Progestogen

Progestogens may be used when cycle disturbances predominate, in benign breast disease and when estrogens are contraindicated. They can control vasomotor symptoms. Progestogens may be used orally or by monthly injection.

Estrogen–Androgen MHT

Androgens reduce hot flushes by direct action at the hypothalamus but are rarely used alone. While estrogen therapy alone may improve libido, women with no improvement after estrogen therapy benefit from the addition of testosterone.

Tibolone

Tibolone is a selective tissue estrogenic activity regulator (STEAR) a completely different kind of MHT. After oral administration, it is rapidly converted into three major substances: two estrogenic, which are responsible for estrogenic effects, and a third with progestogenic and androgenic properties. Tissue-specific effects are due to the interaction of several mechanisms that depend on the target tissue. Tibolone has favourable effects on vasomotor symptoms, vagina, mood and sexual wellbeing and bone but, due to the progestogen like metabolite, does not stimulate the endometrium or breast. At the recommended daily oral dose, tibolone alleviates hot flushes, sleeplessness and fatigue and suppresses elevated FSH levels. Since there is little effect on the endometrium, there is no indication for co-medication with a progestogen.

How Do You Match the Type of MHT to Your Individual Need?

In a Woman with a Uterus

- **Menopause transition and menopause less than one year**
  o Sequential combined regime: Continuous estrogen and cyclical progestogen 12–14 days each month
  o Low dose contraceptive pill if not contraindicated
- **Post-menopause**
  o Continuous combined: Continuous estrogen and progestogen
  o Tibolone

- **Premature ovarian insufficiency**
  - Standard or high-dose estrogen and cyclical or continuous progestogens
  - Low-dose contraceptive pill if not contraindicated
  - Tibolone

In a Woman without a Uterus

- **At any time before or after menopause**
  - Continuous estrogen alone
  - Tibolone

Local Treatment in GSM

  - Oral estriol
  - Vaginal estriol cream
  - Vaginal conjugated estrogen cream

What Are the Different Estrogen and Progestogens Used for MHT?

Minimum effective dose is the principle to be followed while prescribing MHT. The type of hormone and potency needed by the woman may change over time. After starting standard-dose therapy, dose can be lowered and maintained accordingly. Low-dose and ultralow-dose therapies are effective in relieving symptoms and maintaining bone mass.

Conjugated Estrogens

Conjugated estrogens are a mixture of natural estrogens. Used orally, they relieve vasomotor and urogenital symptoms effectively, resulting in a normal vaginal environment within a week. A daily dose of 0.625 mg arrests bone loss. Vaginal application of conjugated estrogens can also be used to treat vaginal dryness and atrophy.

Estriol

Estriol is a natural estrogen particularly effective in relieving the urogenital symptoms related to menopause. It is administered in a dose of 2 mg per day for a few weeks, and then reduced to a dose of 1 mg. Estriol can also be applied with a vaginal applicator as a cream daily for a few weeks followed by a twice-weekly dose.

Estradiol

Estradiol is the most potent natural estrogen available. A dose of 1–2 mg is administered cyclically and adjusted to a minimal effective dose. Continuous preparations use estrogens and progestogens in a fixed dose to avoid bleeding, by combining estradiol with a progestogen.

Progestogens

Progestogens are synthetic forms of progesterone developed because progesterone could not be absorbed orally. The progestogens used for MHT are dydrogestrone, medroxyprogesterone acetate and levonorgestrel. Micronized progesterone is now available and preferred and may be safer than synthetic progestogens. While dydrogestrone and medroxyprogesterone acetate are used orally, micronized progesterone can be used orally or vaginally. Besides this levonorgestrel can be used as an intrauterine device and etonogestrol as an implant.

What are the Non-Oral Delivery Systems for MHT?

Non-oral hormone delivery systems bypass the liver, directly delivering into the blood stream. Direct delivery has a neutral effect on triglycerides, CRP and sex hormone-binding globulin and is preferable for use in women with obesity, glucose intolerance, hypertriglyceridemia, high risk of deep-vein thrombosis and in tobacco users.

Transdermal Delivery by Gel

Gels or cream applications on the skin are convenient and better suited for women living in warm climate who want to use the transdermal route, since local skin reaction from patches are troublesome. Cyclic progestogens are a mandatory adjunct to transdermal therapy in women with an intact uterus.

Transdermal Delivery by Patch

A skin patch is used to deliver estradiol through the skin in a continuous release of a low dose. Contemporary patches now have estradiol incorporated in the glue matrix to minimize skin reactions. The patch is available in three doses, delivering 25, 50 and 100 µg over twenty-four hours. The patch is placed on the hairless skin over the buttock and fixed by palm pressure for five to ten seconds. It is waterproof and stays in position for three to four days.

Transvaginal Administration

Estrogens are reported to effectively combat urogenital symptoms with an 8 mg vaginal dose of estradiol, that is, a mere 10–15 per cent of the dose necessary to alleviate hot flushes and other climacteric disturbances. Progestogen supplementation for endometrial protection is not needed along with the use of vaginal estrogen.

Intrauterine Release

Compared to cyclic oral therapy, a levonorgestrel IUD is more effective in controlling endometrial proliferation and avoiding the erratic bleeding induced by progestogens.

What are the Non-Conventional Options to MHT?

Phytoestrogens

Many women hesitate to continue MHT for more than a few months due to concerns regarding their potential side effects. Therefore, alternative methods of treatment are often sought and easily accepted. Foods of plant origin contain phytoestrogens, which are bioactive compounds that are not normally considered as nutrients but which have possible benefits to human health.

Phytoestrogens exert an estrogenic and antiestrogenic effect due to their similarity in structure to estrogens. A growing body of literature suggests that there are health benefits of phytoestrogens.

There are five major classes of phytoestrogens:

- Isoflavones

- Flavanols
- Flavones
- Flavanones
- Lignans

Isoflavones have emerged as the most interesting class of phytoestrogens as they have an extensive range of biological action. They are found predominantly in legumes, soya milk, tofu and beans. Isoflavones can bind to estrogen receptors just as estrogen. Phytoestrogens have more affinity for estrogen receptors found in the brain, the bones, the bladder and the blood vessels. In some tissues, they have an anti-estrogenic action, blocking the receptor and thereby the action of the endogenous estrogen and its negative effects on the breasts and the uterine lining. They also are cancer enzyme inhibitors by their action on the enzyme tyrosine kinase that promotes cancer-cell growth and their antioxidant effect preventing free radical damage to deoxyribonucleic acid (DNA).

Bioidentical Hormone Therapy

Bioidentical hormone therapy (BHT) is a poorly defined term, commonly used to describe compounded hormone preparations which contain mixtures of various hormones, including estradiol, estrone, estriol, progesterone, testosterone and DHEA, usually prepared by compounding pharmacies. These are not subjected to the same rigorous manufacturing standards, quality control and regulatory oversight as pharmaceutical-grade registered products.

Proponents of BHT often claim, erroneously, that their preparations are made to meet individual needs of women, based on blood or salivary hormone levels. This concept is scientifically flawed, as the ratios of estrone and estriol to the parent estradiol in the body remain relatively constant and it is futile for doctors to write prescriptions for all three hormones in an attempt to do what the body does naturally.

All mainstream clinical and regulatory bodies in women's health advise against the use of these products due to the lack of quality control and regulatory oversight associated with these products, together with lack of evidence of safety and efficacy. Women requesting compounded BHT should be encouraged to consider regulated products containing hormones that are structurally identical to those produced in the body. These are available in a wide range of doses and delivery methods.

How Long Can MHT Be Taken?

The safety of MHT largely depends on age and time since menopause. Healthy women younger than sixty years should not be unduly concerned about the safety profile of MHT. There are no reasons to place mandatory limitations on the duration of MHT and evidence supports safe use for up to five years in healthy women who initiate treatment before sixty years of age.

- In POI, MHT can be prescribed up to the natural age of menopause, further continuation of therapy being a shared decision between the woman and the physician according to the indication and the need.
- In natural menopause, there is safety data for estrogen progestogen use up to five years and for estrogen use up to seven years. Further extended use of MHT is a

Figure 15: Individualization of MHT dosing

MHT dosing

Estrogen / day	Low E	Moderate E	High E
Conjugated estrogen *Premarin*	0.3 mg	0.625 mg	1.25 mg
Estradiol *Progynova, Valest, E V Tab*	0.5 mg	1 mg	2 mg
Transdermal gel *Estogel, Sandrena*	0.5 mg	1 mg	2 mg
Transdermal patch *Estraderm MX, Evorel*	25 µg	50 µg	100 µg

Progestogen sequential daily for 10 to 14 days / month

Dydrogesterone *Duphaston, Dydrogest,* *Dydrofem, Zuviston*	5 mg	10 mg	10 mg
Micronized progesterone *Naturogest, Susten, Gestofit,* *Microgest*	100 mg	200 mg	200 mg
Medroxy progesterone acetate *Deviry, Meprate, Modus*	5 mg	10 mg	10 mg

Progestogen continuous daily dose

Dydrogesterone *Duphaston, Dydrogest,* *Dydrofem, Zuviston*	5 mg	5 - 10 mg	5 - 10 mg
Micronized progesterone *Naturogest, Susten, Gestofit,* *Microgest*	100 mg	100 mg	100 mg
Medroxy progesterone acetate *Deviry, Meprate, Modus*	2.5 mg	2.5 - 5 mg	2.5 - 5 mg
Drosperinone *Dronis*	0.5 mg	-	-
LNG-IUD *Mirena, Eloira*	device releasing 20 µg/24 hours		

Combined OC pills with drosperinone

Ethinyl estradial *Yaz, Dronis 20, Crisanta LS*	20 µg		
Ethinyl estradial *Yasmin, Dronis 30, Crisanta*		30 µg	

Tibolone alone continuous daily

Tibolone *Livial, Tibofem, Tibomax*	2.5 mg daily		

shared decision between the woman and her doctor and may be considered in cases of recurrence of symptoms after stopping therapy and in case of management of osteoporosis when other therapies are contraindicated.

Stopping MHT may be abrupt, or the dose and duration may be tapered off gradually.

Part Three

Part Two

16

The Hormone-Transformation Diet

'Let food be thy medicine, thy medicine shall be thy food.'
—Hippocrates

My Hormonal Harmony Journey

Growing up, I was a child with puppy fat. This continued into my college years and of course, when boys came on the scene, the desire to lose my chubbiness and look attractive was paramount. I went on an exclusively banana and milk diet (in those days, I was not vegan) for a month. After this, I was always on a yo-yo diet and I must have been through five dieticians, each with their own theories. Each one dished out a calorie-based approach with little information on diet and fermentation. While the

289

various diets did help me lose weight, they did not help with my digestion. Subsequently, I ended up with a weak back and a slipped disk. The foundation I laid for my body in my early twenties resulted in a host of 'gut issues' that would take me the next fifteen years of my life to resolve. The one thing I was always proud of were my flat washboard abs. But then in my forties, my waist started getting this strange thickness and those washboard abs slipped into oblivion. I felt like a Renaissance woman in an old Rubenesque painting—voluptuous and beautiful, but fat nonetheless. I knew, being in the field that I am in, that stress along with hormonal changes were contributing to this change in my body shape. My Ayurvedic doctor kept saying it was perimenopause. I seemed to have hit a metabolic wall and my pre-midlife state was holding on to fat to save me. I am glad it gave me the chance to come up with this 'Hormone-Transformation Diet' and the chance to share the knowledge with you.

For women struggling with weight loss issues around this time, I would like to say this before moving on:

- *Make peace with this process and this phase of your life.*
- *Accept the changes that will unfold.*
- *Exercise. Don't go easy on yourself and give this up.*
- *If there is a time to change your relationship with foods, this is it.*
- *Establish a rhythm and routine to your life.*
- *Stop consuming refined sugars.*

Fortunately, in my early thirties, I came under the care of Dr Raveendran, the Ayurvedic genius of India. I also started my study of macrobiotics. I was my own guinea pig, practising on myself the principles of macrobiotic diet between all four levels of my study.

Here is what I did: I finally started paying attention to my body and its intuitive wisdom. While studying macrobiotics, I went cold turkey on foods (which you will learn about in the following chapters) and beverages that did not work for me. I was determined to resolve my digestion, strengthen my gut and get rid of candida. I studied several experts on diet and women's health issues in my quest and since I wanted to live a life free of dietary fads, I focused on the actual 'energy' of foods along with the macrobiotic approach (even with cooking via my catering service for people with hormonal issues). This worked for me and for many of my clients, giving me a 360-degree perspective. I understood the role of estrogen and how it is deeply connected to all facets of a woman's being, not only her weight. With this understanding, I came up with my own unique 'Hormone-Transformation Diet', allowing me to care not only for women with hormonal imbalance in their younger years, but also those in their perimenopause as they headed towards menopause. The core principle of the approach I follow (macrobiotics) is strengthening the gut microbiome to aid detoxification, help in burning fat and restoring the gut-brain axis.

The Hormone-Transformation Diet will touch all you women out there with or without hormone

> *issues. It's a one-size-fits-all approach, which is the uniqueness of this dietary plan. The source list for products mentioned in the transformation diet is available at soulfoodshonali.com.*
>
> *Shonali Sabherwal*

Apart from the fact that a variety of hormones need to be addressed for women's health—estrogen, progesterone, androgens, cortisol and thyroid—there are two organs in particular that need to be functioning well. The first is your gut and the second is your liver.

Your Gut

You need to have a strong gut microbiome to help you process estrogen. Sara Gottffried, a pioneer in the field of hormones, stresses on the need for women to ask their doctors questions about estrobolome, the subset of the microbiome that is essential in metabolizing estrogen.

In the vision I have for the future of personalized functional medicine, this would be the kind of question women would ask their doctors and not get silenced with an eye-roll. As we know, estrogen levels and metabolites are recognized as a causal factor in the etiology of breast cancer. How our estrobolome metabolizes estrogens could explain the reason why some women get breast cancers and others don't.[*]

Estrogen is broken down in the liver. These breakdown products called metabolites are then excreted into the gut

---

[*] Gottfried Sara via Instagram, @saragottfriedmd.

via bile or in the urine. The metabolites that end up in the intestines can be reverted to their original form by certain gut bacteria that produce an enzyme called beta glucuronidase. This allows for estrogen to re-enter the blood stream and be further recycled by the body. Estrogen is meant to be used and then disposed of; therefore, this process of recycling estrogen increases the level circulating in the bloodstream, leading to an overall increase in the risk of developing estrogen-dependent cancers, such as breast and endometrial cancer. We need to follow the golden rule of estrogen—use it, then lose it. So, your diet needs to address the fact that the build-up of estrogen needs clearing almost daily.

Your Liver

The Hormone-Transformation Diet will also focus on your liver. Why? Because, over time, the liver can get lethargic, and when given the right inputs, the liver, in conjunction, with a strong gut, will help detoxify all that extra estrogen. We do not want too much sugar in your blood since this could make your liver listless. What we need instead are vitamins, minerals and the right amino acids to support liver detoxification.

Phases of the Hormone-Transformation Diet

Phase 1. Detoxification over One Week

Consider this phase a detox phase. While you are going through it, you need to keep your bowels moving. Two things that can help at this point are 'detoxing your liver' for a day and 'deworming' yourself to aid the gut. Besides this, continue with your diet as is.

- *Detoxify your liver by taking Triphala.* Not only is it an antioxidant, which will neutralize free radicals, but it aids the liver to cleanse and addresses the gut. Take 1 teaspoon or a tablet twice a day after meals.
- *Support liver detoxification.* Add magnesium citrate 800 mg a day and vitamin C 500 mg to protect the liver cells from any toxins.
- *Deworm using Krimishodhini.* Take one tablet for four days at bedtime while continuing with your current diet plan as is. Add psyllium husk 1 tablespoon at bedtime in a glass of water. You may also take a deworming medication such as albendazole.
- *Add a good probiotic.* Econorm one sachet, Enterogermina one vial or VSl-3 one capsule twice a day.

Phase 2. Elimination of Inflammatory Foods over Two Weeks

The top ten foods that need to be eliminated from your diet for two weeks during Phase 2 are listed below. These may be added back after two weeks but minimized in the long run. Besides these ten foods, you may continue with your diet as is.

1. Sugars, artificial sweeteners, jaggery, maple syrup, agave syrup, brown rice syrup, molasses, date syrup, honey, fruit juices, any food off the shelf having sugars or sugar alcohols like maltitol, sorbitol, xylitol, erythritol, mannitol, lactitol, isomalt and high-fructose-corn syrup.
2. Dairy and dairy products, including yogurt, cheese, paneer, cream, casein, whey protein. Milk includes A2 quality milk as well.
3. Refined oils.

4. Caffeine whether its coffee or tea, Indian chai or any other tea with caffeine, including green tea.
5. Some starchy vegetables which include potato, sweet potato and corn.
6. Citrus fruits like oranges, grapefruit, malta and kinu.
7. Red meat, chicken, eggs and fish.
8. Alcohol of all kinds, including wine.
9. Processed foods. These include foods out of a box like cookies, dried snacks (farsaan) and packaged foods.
10. All grains, including brown rice and millets.

    When you eliminate these pro-inflammatory foods from your diet, the body shifts to a new level so expect to have symptoms of a small detox. They could be in the form of headaches, body odour, irritability, frustration, lethargy, maybe a UTI or a skin issue; it could be anything, as old foods are being discharged from your system. Just hydrate and power on!

Phase 3. The Hormone-Transformation Diet Foods over Three Months

A macrobiotic diet is high in fibre, hence it collects the unwanted estrogen, getting it ready for excretion. Increased dietary fibre will not only lower estrogen build-up, it will also improve the ability of the liver to clear out the excess estrogen.

The top ten foods that need to be added to your diet diet over the three months in Phase 3 are listed below. Most of these foods are immune-boosters and anti-inflammatory.

1. Vegetables, including beetroot, carrots, red pumpkin (lal kaddu or bhopla), turnip (shalgam), peas and other local and seasonal vegetables.

Stress on cruciferous vegetables like cauliflower, broccoli, cabbage, brussels sprouts, radish, mustard, kale. Indole-3-carbinol is a powerful antioxidant found in cruciferous vegetables, which will help metabolize estrogen excess. Sulforaphane is a natural compound found in this group of vegetables. It is activated by myrosinase enzymes—vegetables must be chopped, cooked and then chewed properly to release active sulforaphane. Since cooking cruciferous vegetables lessens their goitrogenic properties, they can be safely had 1–2 times a week by women with thyroid disease.

2. Whole grains, including brown, red or black rice and all millets (specially foxtail millet). Use is restricted to about 150 grams of the cooked grain a day.

3. Beans or lentils, choosing any type of whole beans or lentils up to one serving a day.

4. Fruits, including all local and seasonal fruits, up to three servings a day.

5. Nuts and seeds, only avoiding peanuts. Have 1 tablespoon of chia seeds and flax seeds a day.

6. Soy in the form of tofu and tempeh may be included 2–3 times a week.

7. Healthy fats including all cold-pressed oils like olive, sesame, coconut, ghee and mustard. Get good fats out of foods like oily fish, walnuts, cashews, pistachios, almonds, avocado, flax, sunflower, pumpkin, sesame and chia seeds, and dark chocolate.

8. Fermented foods including miso, sauerkraut, pressed salads, kimchi, kefir and buttermilk with 3–4 servings of these foods daily and between meals.

9. Fish, meat and eggs may be included in your diet after one month. Try to stay with white lean meats, not cured

meats. An egg a day with both white and yolk is also permitted.

10. Sweeteners, including brown rice syrup, agave, pure maple, stevia, xylitol, manuka honey and organic jaggery, may be included after two months. Restrict these to twice a week.

A hormone-boosting water infusion made with the following ingredients can be had through the day in all three phases:

- Juice of one lemon
- Pinch of red chilli powder
- Slice of ginger (optional)
- Pinch of fresh turmeric powder
- Half teaspoon of cinnamon powder
- Five cups water

Bring to a boil and then simmer for ten minutes. Cool it and drink the infusion through the day.

The Hormone-Transformation Diet

Here are sample diet plans for the two main phases—the Elimination phase and the Hormone-Transformation Diet phase.

Phase 2. Elimination Phase (Two Weeks)

Check and start implementing the foods to eliminate. This is a plant-based diet week, so please keep it that way. In the Elimination Phase:

- Try and stick with the initial phase of no grain for two weeks. The guidelines for this are outlined in the section on outcomes and adjustments.
- Do not skip any meal.
- The Hormone-Transformation Smoothie is a must daily.
- If you experience gas or feel bloated with beetroot kanji, then try it out for one more day. If you still don't adjust to it, then switch to buttermilk
- For those with hypertension, exchange the kanji with buttermilk.
- If you feel hungry in the evening, then add a fruit (that is, if you do not do the Hormone-Transformation Smoothie).
- You can choose your preferred cooking style so long as you include the foods specified in the diet.

Day 1

Breakfast (8–9 a.m.)

Tofu scrambled or mixed vegetable scrambled with sprouts (cooked)

Mid-Morning (10–11 a.m.)

Beetroot kanji or buttermilk (150 ml)

Lunch (1–2 p.m.)

Refried beans or green mung dal (cooked) in lettuce wraps (4) with green salad

Evening (4–5 p.m.)

Hormone Harmony Smoothie (choose any one from the recipe section)

Dinner (6.30 p.m. to 7.30 p.m.)

Lentil Soup with vegetables

Day 2

Breakfast (8 a.m.)

Sprouted green mung bowl cooked to your style

Mid-morning (10–11 a.m.)

Beetroot kanji or buttermilk (150 ml)

Lunch (1–2 p.m.)

Chickpea cutlets (2) with salsa

Evening (4–5 p.m.)

Hormone Harmony Smoothie (choose any one)

Dinner (6.30 p.m. to 7.30 p.m.)

Falafel with avocado, tomato and red onion salsa

Day 3

Breakfast (8 a.m.)

Lentil pancake (chilla) with chutney

Mid-morning (10–11 a.m.)

Beetroot kanji or buttermilk (150 ml)

Lunch (1–2 p.m.)

Red salad with beetroot, red cabbage and harissa dressing

Evening (4–5 p.m.)

Hormone Harmony Smoothie (choose any one)

Dinner (6.30 p.m. to 7.30 p.m.)

Carrot lentil soup with almond bread or almond flour roti (Indian flatbread)

Day 4

Breakfast (8 a.m.)

Lentil idli with coconut chutney

Mid-Morning (10–11 a.m.)

Beetroot kanji or buttermilk (150 ml)

Lunch (1–2 p.m.)

Tofu and black bean stir fry (omit tofu if you do not want
to eat it)

Evening (4–5 p.m.)

Hormone Harmony Smoothie (choose any one)

Dinner (6.30 p.m. to 7.30 p.m.)

Pumpkin soup with sprouts (puree)

Day 5

Breakfast (8 a.m.)

Lentil dosa with coconut chutney

Mid-morning (10–11 a.m.)

Beetroot kanji or buttermilk (150 ml)

Lunch (1–2 p.m.)

Italian lentil salad

Evening (4–5 p.m.)

Hormone Harmony Smoothie (choose any one)

Dinner (6.30 p.m. to 7.30 p.m.)

Tandoori tofu kebabs with cashew paste raita

Day 6

Breakfast (8 a.m.)

Fruit porridge with seed granola

Mid-morning (10–11 a.m.)

Beetroot kanji or buttermilk (150 ml)

Lunch (1–2 p.m.)

Val (white beans) in a coconut curry and flaxseed roti (Indian flatbread)

Evening (4–5 p.m.)

Hormone Harmony Smoothie (choose any one)

Dinner (6.30 p.m. to 7.30 p.m.)

Beetroot soup with lemon zest

Day 7

Breakfast (8 a.m.)

Cooked sprouts with vegetables

Mid-morning (10–11 a.m.)

Beetroot kanji or buttermilk (150 ml)

Lunch (1–2 p.m.)

Sesame seed curry with black chana sprouts

Evening (4–5 p.m.)

Hormone Harmony Smoothie (choose any one)

Dinner (6.30 p.m. to 7.30 p.m.)

Sweet potato with broccoli salad

Phase 3. The Hormone-Transformation Diet (Three Months)

While following this plan, you will add 1 tablespoon of a fermented food at lunch and dinner from the fermentation section of the recipe chapter.

You can now add 125 gm of cooked, gluten-free grains in a day:

- Brown, red or black rice
- Sorghum (jovar)
- Foxtail millet (kangni)
- Proso (cheena)
- Barnyard (sanwa)
- Buckwheat (kuttu)
- Finger millet (ragi)—cooler climate

- Pearl millet (bajra)—cooler climate
- Amaranth (rajgeera) and quinoa are pseudo-grains from the family of grasses

Barley (pearl millet), whole wheat (daliya or bulgur), all-purpose flour (maida), couscous and semolina (sooji) are not considered gluten-free grains. Tapioca pearls (sabudana) is a starch and cannot be included in any phase.

If you feel bloated, lethargic and experience sugar cravings, it means that you are far more sensitive to carbohydrates. In this case revert back to the first phase (where you eliminated grain) for one more week.

Listed here is a model seven-day plan for the Hormone-Transformation Diet. It gives you plenty of options for breakfast and entrées from different cuisines, which you can access in the recipe section. In the charts are listed vegetarian and non-vegetarian option for meals. The letter V signifies vegetarian, VV vegetarian vegan and NV non-vegetarian. Also, in the chart are identified Indian or Western formats. You can swap lunch and dinner meals but limit grain carbohydrates to those specified.

	Menu	Meal type	Cuisine
Day 1			
Breakfast	Scrambled eggs	NV	Western
	Blushing papaya and banana smoothie	VV	Western
	Millet upma or poha	V	Indian
Mid-morning	Kanji or buttermilk		
Lunch	Curried lentils with carrots and peas	VV	Indian

	Asian salmon and brown rice	NV	Pan-Asian
Evening snack	Hormone harmony smoothie Choose any one	VV	Western
Dinner	Tofu vindaloo and grain	VV	Indian
	Chicken vindaloo and grain	NV	Indian
Day 2			
Breakfast	Easy egg white omelette	NV	Western
	Any one smoothie	VV	Western
	Millet porridge	VV	Western
Mid-morning	Kanji or buttermilk		
Lunch	Qunioa tabbouleh	VV	Middle-eastern
	Non-vegetarians add meat of choice	NV	
	Red rice, urad dal and lauki in tomatoes	V	Indian
Evening snack	Hormone harmony smoothie	VV	Western
	Choose any one		
Dinner	Mushroom moussaka with sweet potato pancakes	VV	Greek
	Non-vegetarians add meat of choice	NV	Greek
Day 3			
Breakfast	Boiled egg with sourdough bread or chapatti	NV	Western
	Any one smoothie	VV	Western
	Red or brown rice poha with vegetables	VV	Indian
Mid-Morning	Kanji or buttermilk		
Lunch	Black bean cutlets with yellow pepper sauce	VV	Western

	Moong sprout pav bhaji with jovar rotis or sourdough bread	V	Indian
Evening Snack	Hormone harmony smoothie Choose any one	VV	Western
Dinner	Middle-Eastern lentils with quinoa and sweet potato pancakes	VV	Middle Eastern
	Non-vegetarians add meat of choice	NV	Middle Eastern
Day 4			
Breakfast	Boiled egg with sourdough bread or chapatti	NV	Western
	Any one smoothie	VV	Western
	Brown rice idli and coconut chutney	V	Indian
Mid-Morning	Kanji or buttermilk		
Lunch	Stir fry tofu and black bean with sourdough bread or jovar rotis	VV	Pan-Asian
	Non-vegetarians can add choice of meat	NV	Pan-Asian
Evening Snack	Hormone harmony smoothie Choose any one	VV	Western
Dinner	Moong stuffed teendas with jovar roti	VV	Indian
	Japanese steamed fish with brown rice	NV	Japanese
	Wild mushroom quinoa pilaf	V	Western
Day 5			
Breakfast	Poached egg with sourdough or amaranth roti (flatbread)	NV	Western
	Any one smoothie	VV	Western

	Brown rice cutlets with chutney	VV	Indian
Mid-Morning	Kanji or buttermilk		
Lunch	Stuffed bell peppers with quinoa	VV	Western
	Non-vegetarians can add choice of meat	NV	Pan-Asian
	Turai with brown rice	V	Indian
Evening Snack	Hormone harmony smoothie Choose any one	VV	Western
Dinner	Buckwheat noodles in ginger broth or buckwheat (kuttu) roti with vegetable or dal of choice	VV	Japanese
	Non-vegetarians can add choice of meat	NV	Japanese
Day 6			
Breakfast	Steel-cut oats savoury or with steamed apples	V	Western Indian
	Any one smoothie	VV	Western
	Buckwheat pancakes with manuka honey	V	Western
Mid-Morning	Kanji or buttermilk		
Lunch	Gado Gado	VV	Indonesian
	Non-vegetarians can add choice of meat	NV	Pan-Asian
	Millet kichari with split green lentils and vegetables	V	Indian
Evening Snack	Hormone harmony smoothie Choose any one	VV	Western
Dinner	Zucchini noodles with basil pesto	VV	Italian

	Non-vegetarians can add choice of meat	NV	
	Stuffed, steamed parwals with jovar rotis	V	Indian
Day 7			
Breakfast	Poached egg with sourdough and avocado	NV	Western
	Any one smoothie	VV	Western
	Besan chilla with chutney Kanji or buttermilk	V	Indian
Mid-Morning	Cauliflower maranca	V	Western
Lunch	Non-vegetarians can add choice of meat	NV	Pan-Asian
	Brown rice cabbage pilaf with yellow lentils	V	Indian
Evening Snack	Hormone harmony smoothie Choose any one	VV	Western
Dinner	Caramelized onions sauce in quinoa pasta with veggies of choice	VV	Italian
	Non-vegetarians can add choice of meat	NV	Italian
	Green mushroom curry with jovar rotis	V	Indian

Outcomes and Adjustments of the Hormone-Transformation Diet

Phase 1 and Phase 2

- Release toxins that play havoc with your hormones.
- Assist this process with a dhaara pizhichil treatment at an Ayurvedic space as an outpatient at this time (optional).

- Add 20–25 gm of cooked grain carbs if you cannot manage a no-grain week. However, it will suit you to keep to no inclusion of grain for at least a week. For women who do intense workouts you could increase this to 35 gm a day.
- For protein consume an average of 100 gm a day. This includes vegan, vegetarian or non-vegetarian protein.
- The goal is to regularize your bowel movements. They need to regularize and be happening daily or show signs of improvement.
- The goal is also to help body to start shedding weight if needed.
- Keep a 12-hour gap between dinner and breakfast.
- Feel free to use any cooking styles and cuisines, as long as you keep within the foods specified and use them.
- Don't drink alcohol.
- Include a sizeable portion of vegetables as specified.
- Try including ½ teaspoon of spirulina or 1 teaspoon of wheatgrass in water to help the liver.
- Use sea, rock or Himalayan pink salt.
- Add 1 tablespoon of flax or chia seeds to this phase.

Phase 3

- The aim of this phase is to help you to cultivate a completely new relationship with food. We hope that the Hormone-Transformation Diet will be your diet for life 80 per cent of the time.
- In this phase you will start adding grains as specified.
- For vegans, you can optimize cooked protein in the following portions included at lunch and dinner: tofu 120 gm, lentils 100 gm, tempeh 80 gm, nuts 32 gm,

seeds 40 gm. Stick to 25 per cent of daily calories of protein consumption.

- Can increase 120–125 gm of cooked grain carbs, spread over three meals or two meals.
- Don't drink alcohol.
- Include healthy fats from coconuts, avocado, cold-pressed oils, nuts, seeds.
- Include a lot of vegetables. Vary cooking styles with the weather and in summers both raw and cooked. (With IBS avoid raw foods.)
- If you feel you are carb-sensitive or insulin resistant, limit the intake of starchy vegetables and focus on all others: cruciferous vegetables (have one these daily), leafy greens and all local and seasonal vegetables.
- Limit fruits to two servings a day.
- Minimize dairy. Cheese lovers may use aged cheese.
- Use sea, rock or Himalayan pink salt.
- Add 1 tablespoon of flax or chia seeds to this phase.
- Adding milk thistle to support the liver will help.
- Get into the habit of using a kitchen weighing scale to measure carbs and protein macros.
- You can cook in any cuisine or use any style of cooking to suit yourself, just as long as you keep to your food groups of grain, protein (vegetarian protein, fish or meats of your choice), vegetables, fermented foods, nuts, seeds and fruit.

Top Ten Snack Options if You Are Hungry

1. Carrot juice, beets and spinach with apple. If desired, add spirulina powder.

2. Fruit with yogurt. Non-dairy option for vegans.
3. Fruit salad with nuts (1 cup).
4. Cucumber, carrot or celery sticks with hummus.
5. Sweet potato baked with coconut cream or hummus or some ghee with toppings.
6. Berries with feta cheese.
7. Boiled egg with avocado.
8. Crispbread or roti (Indian flatbread) with organic raw peanut or almond butter.
9. Mock egg tofu salad with roti (Indian flatbread).
10. Sweet potato boiled or steamed and cubed with Indian chaat masala.

Following up the Hormone-Transformation Diet

To maintain the benefits of the Hormone-Transformation Diet you can gradually introduce foods that you avoided or eliminated over the three-month and two-week period of your transformation. While watching your digestion is the key, when you go back to the following foods you may notice symptom manifestations to which you may now be sensitized with your new-found understanding. Here are some of the other conversations your body will have with you.

Foods That You May Cheat With	Symptoms They May Manifest
Dairy	Bloating, gas, acid reflux, diarrhoea, constipation, lethargy, foggy thinking or allergies

Sugar, sweeteners, including all-purpose flour (maida)	Crazy thoughts, anxiety, craving more sugar, irritability, anger, fatigue, stomach distension or insomnia
Wheat and gluten	Distension, gas, bloating, acid reflux, fatigue, joint pain, lethargy, puffiness, headaches or allergies
Citrus fruits	Watery eyes, mucus, headaches and acid reflux
Refined oil	Heaviness, mucus, lethargy, irritability or a craving for salt
Animal foods (specifically red meat)	Constipation, slower digestion and heat produced in the body
Table salt	Contracted and tight condition, fatigue, craving for water and sugar and refined flour
Hard baked and roasted snacks (farsaan)	Same symptoms as salt and in addition aggravated joint pains (arthritis), dense/dark thought processes, slower digestion and aggravated acid reflux
Commercial foods with additives preservatives	Crave sugar, aggravate digestion, irritability, anger, aggravate lung-related conditions, create mucus and promote negative thoughts

| **FOOD HABITS** THAT CAUSE HORMONES TO GO OFF BALANCE | SHORT- AND LONG-TERM IMPACT |
WHAT ARE THE CONSEQUENCES	
Bad quality fats—trans fats, refined oils, hydrogenated fat, sugar: which includes jaggery and brown sugar, refined white flour (maida), whole wheat (gluten), cured meat and chicken with growth hormones.	Dementia, Alzheimer's, brain-related issues, ADHD, insulin resistance, PCOS, obesity, diabetes, cancer, heart disease
Increased cravings Blood sugar imbalances High CRP (C-reactive protein) which is an inflammatory marker	
Dairy, from cows given growth hormones, antibiotics, the contraceptive pill and any steroids	Risk of getting cancers - usually estrogen driven: breast, uterine and cervical
Increased growth hormone Imbalance in estrogen and progesterone	
Lack of fibre in the diet	Heart disease, cancer, PCOS, insulin resistance
Blood sugar imbalances Increased cravings Bad digestive habits Weight and Obesity Toxic estrogen build-up	
Sugar-free products, artificial sweeteners, this includes high-fructose corn syrup	Cravings in-between meals, PCOS, insulin resistance, increase in fat
Increased cravings Blood sugar imbalances Weight gain Insulin resistance	
Excessive Alcohol	Low testosterone, PCOS, insulin resistance, increased fat
Increased cravings Estrogen dominance	

HABITS THAT CAUSE HORMONES TO GO OFF BALANCE WHAT ARE THE CONSEQUENCES	SHORT- AND LONG-TERM IMPACT
Avoiding breakfast Cravings Binge-eating Leptin/Ghrelin resistance Increased cortisol Hypothyroid	Weight gain Diabetes Increase in wrong carbs consumption
Late-night snacking & overeating Blood sugar imbalances Sleeplessness and insomnia Decrease in growth hormone Increased cortisol	Lack of concentration and focus Poor sleep impacting stress Weight Anxiety
Yo-Yo dieting and prolonged fasting, leading to low calorific diet Hypothyroid Increase in cortisol	Binge eating Decrease in metabolism Weight
Lack of balance in protein, carbohydrates and fats Blood sugar imbalances Increase in cortisol Increased cravings	Cravings in-between meals, PCOS, insulin resistivity, diabetes, cancer, obesity, dementia
Emotional-stressful eating Blood sugar imbalances Increase in cortisol Increased cravings	Binge eating, insulin resistance, weight

Indian cooking on high heat with refined oils	Leaky gut, autoimmune disease, insulin imbalances, diabetes, weight gain, Alzheimer's disease, gut-brain axis issues
Inflammation High CRP (C-reactive protein)	

The Ten Steps towards a Healthier Kitchen

You should work to clear your kitchen of all dangerous material, including xenoestrogens (hormone depleters) to which you can be exposed to by contact or ingestion. The use of the following items, materials and utensils is best avoided, minimized or scrapped completely:

1. Aluminium and Teflon cookware. Replace them with stainless steel or cast-iron utensils.
2. Detergents with chemicals and any materials that mimic estrogen. Replace with eco-friendly cleaners and detergents.
3. Plastic use, exposure to BPA (bisphenols), plastic clingwrap, containers, bottles and bags. Buy glass storage containers.
4. Styrofoam containers.
5. Food products with artificial sweeteners.
6. Products with high-fructose-corn syrup.
7. Products with preservatives and food colours.
8. Cured meats or animal food (which have dioxins which alter thyroid function).
9. Flame retardants used in coating kitchen cabinets.
10. Foods that have BHA used as gum for preservation.

17

Recipes

'Start where you are. Use what you have. Do what you can.'

—Arthur Ashe

Mandatory Smoothies in Phase 2

Hormone Harmony Smoothie #1
1 scoop of vegan protein powder
1 scoop of greens powder or 1 cup of any leafy greens
1 tablespoon of flaxseed oil
1 cup almond milk or milk substitute
¼ cup berries or any fruit
1 scoop inulin powder
Blend all ingredients together.

Hormone Harmony Smoothie #2
1 serving of a vegan protein blend

2 tablespoons of chia or flax seeds
1 cup almond milk or milk substitute
1 tablespoon of any good nut butter
1 scoop inulin powder
Blend all ingredients together.

Hormone Harmony Smoothie #3

1 serving of a vegan protein blend
2 tablespoons of chia or flax seeds
1 cup almond milk or milk substitute
¼ cup berries (or any seasonal fruit)
1 scoop inulin powder
Blend all ingredients together.

Hormone Harmony Smoothie #4

1 cup kale or any leafy green (not spinach)
½ banana and ½ apple
1 tablespoon walnuts
4 mint leaves
2 one-inch pieces of cucumber
1 cup coconut water
1 tablespoon chia seeds
Blend all ingredients together.

Additional Smoothies and Juices in Phase 3

Strawberry-Kissed Banana Smoothie

2 servings
2/3 cup yogurt or soy yogurt
1½ cup coconut milk
1 teaspoon chia seeds
2 bananas and 2 cups strawberries

Blend all the above ingredients until creamy.

Banana Bliss and Pineapple Smoothie
1 cup cubed pineapple
1 medium banana (chopped)
7 strawberries (optional)
1 cup yogurt or dairy free yogurt
1 teaspoon vanilla extract (optional)
1 teaspoon flax seeds
Some ice cubes
Blend all the above ingredients until smooth. Garnish with mint.

Grapes and Green Juice
2 servings
15 grapes (any, preferably red)
4 celery sticks with leaves chopped 4 inches
Some ice cubes
Blend all the above ingredients until smooth.

Blushing Papaya and Banana Smoothie
2 servings
1 banana cut into sizeable chunks
½ papaya cut into sizeable chunks
½ cup soy yogurt
1 teaspoon spirulina (optional)
Blend all the above ingredients until creamy.

Gorgeous Greens Smoothie
2 servings
1 apple chopped
½ cup water or vegetable stock
1 cup of sprouts

1 tablespoon spirulina powder
2 teaspoons lemon juice
1 teaspoon of wheat grass powder
4 tablespoons aloe vera juice
½ teaspoon of cumin powder
Blend all the above ingredients until smooth.

Mixed Fruit and Berry Smoothie
2 servings
½ cup berries
2 tablespoon pomegranate seeds
1 tablespoon sunflower or pumpkin seeds (unsalted)
1 teaspoon flax seeds
1 apple
½ papaya or 1 mango (if in season)
½ teaspoon of wheat grass powder
½ cup coconut milk
Blend all the above ingredients and pour over ice.

Antioxidant Pomegranate Stress Buster
2 servings
2 pomegranates
Some ice
1 teaspoon chia seeds
Blend all the above ingredients and pour over ice.

Breakfast Recipes

Millet Upma/Poha
4 servings
1 cup barnyard or kodo millet or cheena millet (yellow foxtail millet for gluten intolerance)
½ cup ghee or any good cold-pressed oil

1 tsp black mustard seeds
1 tsp cumin seeds
1 pinch hing (preferably organic)
5 curry leaves fresh or dried
1 small green chilli, chopped fine
1 small onion chopped fine
½ teaspoon rock or sea salt
Coconut, cilantro or curry leaves for garnish
3 cups water

1. Roast the millet in a dry pan over medium heat until slightly brown. Set aside in a bowl to cool. Boil in 1½ cup water. Keep aside.
2. Heat a saucepan on medium heat and add oil or ghee, then the mustard and cumin seeds. When the seeds pop, add the other spices except the salt.
3. Stir in the onions, cilantro and chilli and cook until onion is browned.
4. Add the salt and water and bring to a boil.
5. Stir in the roasted kodo or millet and let it boil for two minutes while stirring continuously to prevent lumps from forming.
6. Turn down the heat and cover. Cook for 5–7 minutes for the millet.
7. Garnish with grated coconut and cilantro.

Yummiest Brown Rice or Millet Porridge
½ cup of leftover brown rice
¼ cup water or almond milk
1 tablespoon of mounaka raisins
½ apple cut into four and sliced thin and long

1 tablespoon walnuts roasted and chopped
1 tablespoon almonds roasted and chopped
Dash of cinnamon

1. Blend cooked brown rice with water or almond milk.
    Don't blend fine keep it grainy.
2. In the meantime, set apples to stew covered with a little
    water and a dash of cinnamon.
3. Put brown rice in a porridge bowl, layer with apples,
    add mounaka raisins and top it with nuts.

Brown Rice or Millet Idlis
Makes 16 idlis
¾ cup brown rice soaked in the morning
¼ cup white urad dhal soaked in the morning

1. Grind both rice and urad dal in the evening and mix
    together.
2. Must be ground extra fine, so not grainy.
3. Ferment overnight.
4. The batter is ready to use the next morning.

Brown Rice Croquettes or Cutlets
Makes 6 croquettes
3 cups of cooked basic brown rice
1 carrot grated
1 onion cut small and fine
3 cloves of garlic chopped fine
3 tablespoons black sesame seeds roasted
½ cup breadcrumbs
½ cup coriander leaves

Sea or rock salt, chilli powder or black pepper powder
1 tablespoon extra-virgin olive oil

1. Sauté carrot, onion and garlic in a pan on a low fire covered for 5 minutes.
2. Mix in with the rice.
3. Shape into 8 croquettes (wet your hands with water while doing this).
4. Mix breadcrumbs and black sesame seeds on a plate.
5. Roll the croquettes so they are coated on both sides.
6. Pan fry in a shallow dish or bake at 150°C for forty minutes on a foil sheet which is oiled.

Soup Recipes

Beetroot Soup with Lemon
4 servings
4 cooked beetroots (pressure cook or steam)
3 cups vegetable stock (non-vegetarians can use chicken stock)
Sea or rock salt to taste
Zest of 2 lemons

1. Steam beetroots, put into a blender.
2. Make vegetable stock.
3. Combine the stock and beetroot and bring back to cook.
4. Before serving, stir in salt and lemon zest

Basic Vegetable Stock for Soups and Curries
Makes 12 cups
4 celery stalks cut small
2 onions diced

4 cloves of garlic peeled and cut small
3–4 carrots cubed
2 cup mushrooms chopped down
A handful of parsley
4 bay leaves (tej patta)
Sea or rock salt
16 cups of water

1. Add onions, garlic and salt in a large vessel, adding 1 cup of water initially. Simmer for ten minutes after the first boil.
2. Add the remaining vegetables to water and bring to a boil.
3. Reduce heat and cook on a low fire for about one hour, so the liquid will boil down to twelve cups.
4. Run water through a sieve, pressing down vegetables to squeeze out water. You can either discard the vegetables or use it in a soup.
5. Use this stock for soups, some vegetable curries and some cold vegetable drinks.

Sweet Miso Soup
12 servings
8 cups water or vegetable stock
1 small squash/red pumpkin (bhopla) cubed
1 medium onion cut into thin rounds
1 small white radish (mooli) cut into thin rounds
6 tablespoons white or barley miso
1 green onion stalk slice fine for garnish

1. Bring eight cups of water to a boil
2. Add onion to the pot. Simmer uncovered for five minutes.

3. Add the radish and simmer another five minutes.
4. Add the squash and simmer until tender about five more minutes. Remove from heat
5. Place small amount of the hot soup in a small bowl, add the miso, whisk until smooth and return to pot.
6. Stir and garnish with green onions.
7. Garnish with parsley
8. Do not boil soup again after adding miso as beneficial micro-organisms get destroyed.

My Moms's Broccoli Soup
4 servings
5 cups of water or vegetable stock
1½ cup chopped broccoli
1 small onion cut really fine
½ sweet potato cubed

1. Bring water, broccoli, sweet potato and onion to a boil (or pressure cook) or use vegetable stock.
2. Cover and simmer ten minutes.
3. After vegetables are tender, cool liquid and put in a blender or use hand blender.
4. Garnish with chopped broccoli.

Fresh Corn Chowder Soup
Makes 6 cups
1 onion diced
2 medium celery stalks chopped fine
6 corns shelled
1 large sweet potato cubed
4 cups vegetable stock or water

1. Place the onion, celery stalks, corn and sweet potatoes in stock or water in a pot.
2. Bring to a boil, reduce heat and simmer covered until potatoes are tender fifteen minutes.
3. Add 1 teaspoon salt and ½ teaspoon black pepper and simmer five minutes more.
4. After cooling, blend in a mixer and return to heat for one more boil.
5. Garnish with parsley or coriander.

Round Vegetable Soup

4 servings
½ cup yam (suran) cubed
2 turnips (shalgam) cubed
4 colocasia (arbi) cut small
2 carrots diced
1 white radish (mooli) cut small
1 onion sliced long and thin
3½ inch cinnamon sticks
4 cloves
1 tablespoon curry powder
1 tablespoon olive oil
3 cups of water or vegetable stock

1. Add oil to a soup pot. Before it heats up add onions, cinnamon and cloves. Sauté until onions get a little soft.
2. Add vegetables in the following order—turnips, yam, colocasia, white radish and carrots. Sauté for ten minutes and then add the curry powder.
3. Add water or stock and after first boil, simmer on low for twenty minutes.

4. As soon as the vegetables are tender, blend with a hand blender.
5. Garnish with parsley.

Tomato Shorba
2 servings
Ingredients
1 cup tomatoes diced
1 cup coconut milk
6 curry leaves
1 teaspoon cumin seeds

1. Add some olive oil to a soup pan.
2. Add cumin seeds and sauté.
3. Add the curry leaves and tomatoes. Sauté for a few minutes.
4. Add the coconut milk and let it come to a boil on slow.
5. Add sea salt in the end and garnish with chopped fresh coriander.

Hearty Brown Rice Soup
6 servings
1 cup chopped onions
1 tablespoon olive oil
1 cup cooked brown rice
Pinch of thyme, marjoram and sea salt
8 cups of vegetable stock or boiling water
1 tablespoon of soy sauce
1 cup cooked chick-peas

1. In a skillet sauté the onions in olive oil over medium heat until translucent.

2. In a large saucepan combine onions with all the rest of the ingredients and bring to a boil. Reduce heat and simmer for five minutes.
3. Blend with a hand blender but save some of the mix before blending and add to the soup pot after blending.

Main Meal Recipes

Stir-Fried Tofu and Black Beans
2 servings
½ cup black rajma (kidney beans)
250 gms of tofu cubed
Small ½ inch piece of ginger, sliced long
2 garlic cloves, minced
2 tablespoons corn, boiled
1 teaspoon toasted sesame oil
2 green onions cut sideways
Sea or rock salt and black pepper

1. Soak black bean overnight and pressure cook next day.
2. Heat oil in wok and fry tofu on either side. Set aside.
3. Add ginger and garlic to the same wok.
4. Add the black beans and corn and stir fry for five minutes on high flame.
5. Add tofu and cook for 2–3 minutes.
6. Season with sea salt and pepper.
7. Garnish with spring onions.

Green Mung Bean Warm Bowl
4 servings
¼ cup green mung, soaked overnight and boiled

1 large carrot grated
½ red bell pepper skinned and diced
1 teaspoon ginger grated
2 tablespoon lemon juice
½ teaspoon mustard seeds
1 small green chilli chopped
10 curry leaves
1 tablespoon coriander leaves
Sea or rock salt to taste

1. Heat oil in a skillet, add mustard seeds and let them pop. When popping stops add chilli, curry leaves and fry for thirty seconds.
2. Mix this in the green mung, add vegetables, coriander leaves and lime.
3. Toss gently before serving.

Mock Egg Tofu Salad
6 servings
250 gm tofu
1 onion grated
2 celery stalks, cut fine
2 carrots grated
Sea or rock salt to taste
1 tablespoon of white wine vinegar

1. Steam the tofu (make sure all the water is squeezed out of your tofu block) and keep aside.
2. Mix all the ingredients and crumble tofu with your hand and mix well.
3. Chill for 10–15 minutes first.
4. Great in a sandwich or on a crackers or by itself.

Refried Beans

8 servings
2 cups cooked red kidney beans (rajma) mashed when warm
2 tablespoons olive oil
2 cups onions, minced
6 garlic pods, minced
1 teaspoon sea salt
Black pepper
1 small green bell pepper, minced

1. Heat olive oil in a skillet, add onions and garlic.
2. Add cumin and salt and sauté for 5–7 minutes until onions are pink.
3. Add bell peppers and black pepper.
4. Turn heat to low and add cooked beans.
5. Cook for about ten minutes until all flavours absorbed.

Greens Salad

4 servings
Any leafy greens in a bunch about 8–10 leaves
1 tablespoon red wine vinegar
1 tablespoon shallots (Madras onions)
½ teaspoon mustard
Sea or rock salt and black pepper
Walnuts (optional)

1. Whisk together the red vinegar, shallots, mustard, salt and black pepper.
2. Toss in with greens.
3. Can add walnuts at the end.

Chickpea Pepperey Salad
4 servings
1 onion diced
1 each of red, yellow and green bell peppers diced
2 cups cooked chick-peas
2 bundles bok choy, cut long and steamed
Olives (optional)
For dressing
¼ cup olive oil
3 tbsp balsamic vinegar
3 garlic cloves minced
Grated zest of 1 lime and juice
Sea or rock salt to taste

1. Get together ingredients in a salad bowl removing the skin of red pepper.
2. For the dressing heat oil add garlic, then remove from heat and whisk in balsamic vinegar and lime juice with zest and salt.
3. Toss the salad and mix dressing.
4. Chill before serving.

Lentil Soup with Vegetables
2 servings
½ cup yellow lentils, pigeon pea (toovar) or channa (gram)
½ teaspoon cumin seeds
½ teaspoon turmeric
½ teaspoon red chilli flakes
1 cup vegetable stock
1 teaspoon cardamom seeds
1 teaspoon mustard seeds
1/2 onion sliced into half moons
1 garlic pod crushed

Sea or rock salt to taste
2 tablespoons of olive oil

1. Pressure cook lentils with cumin, chilli flakes and puree once done.
2. Heat oil in a pan, add mustard and cardamom seeds and fry until they pop.
3. Add the onion and garlic and cook until it browns a bit.
4. Mix in with the lentils and give it a stir.
5. Once lentil soup is ready add salt to taste.

Quinoa Tabbouleh

2 servings
½ cup quinoa
2 green onions cut sideways
1 tomato
½ cup boiled peas
Fistful of parsley
Fistful of coriander
2 tablespoons walnuts (optional)
Dressing
3 tablespoons extra virgin olive oil
1 teaspoon Dijon mustard
2 garlic pods, crushed
Juice of ½ lime
Sea or rock salt and black pepper to taste

1. Prepare quinoa by rinsing thoroughly and boiling in one cup of water.
2. When quinoa is done add the chopped vegetables, coriander and parsley.
3. Mix together gently.

4. Mix in salad dressing.
5. Toast walnuts in a pan, chop roughly (after cooling) and toss into the tabbouleh.

Mushroom Moussaka

8 servings
3 medium eggplants, peeled or as is
2 cups of onions chopped
Sea or rock salt to taste
2 tablespoons of olive oil or ghee
1 kilo of mushrooms chopped
5 pods of garlic minced
¾ cup tomato puree
2 cups of tomatoes chopped
1 teaspoon cinnamon
Black pepper to taste
1 cup parsley
1 teaspoon of oregano
1 teaspoon of basil
2 tablespoons olive oil

1. Slice eggplants into round slices, salt them on either side and set aside for twenty minutes.
2. Dry eggplant after twenty minutes with a kitchen towel.
3. Oil a baking tray. Preheat oven to 190°C.
4. Place eggplant on a baking tray and bake for twenty-five minutes
5. Heat olive oil in a pan, add onions and salt and cook for a while on medium heat. Stir until the onions change their colour to pink.
6. Add mushrooms and stir for about ten minutes.
7. Add tomatoes, tomato puree, cinnamon, oregano, basil and pepper.

8. Bring to a slow boil and let it simmer uncovered for fifteen minutes.
9. Remove from the heat and stir in parsley.

Asian Salmon with Brown Rice
2 servings
1 inch piece of ginger
2 garlic cloves, minced
½ carrot sliced thinly
2 ½ cups mushrooms, sliced
2 tablespoons coriander, chopped
2 teaspoons honey
2 fish steaks (any)
1 tsp Chinese 5 spice powder
1 tbsp soy sauce

Chinese 5 spice powder
1 teaspoon of pepper (schezwan pepper preferred)
1 teaspoon of ground star anise
1 teaspoon ground fennel seeds
½ teaspoon ground cloves
½ teaspoon ground cinnamon
½ teaspoon sea salt
¼ teaspoon white pepper
Combine all the ingredients after dry roasting and grind together or stay whole

1. Marinate the fish (after washing) in the Chinese 5 spice powder by smearing on either side of the fish steaks.
2. Steam or broil the fish steaks for ten minutes, turn each side when half-way done.
3. Heat a pan, add soy sauce, ginger, garlic, ginger, honey, carrots and warm through for 4–5 minutes. Add mushrooms and sauté for 2–3 minutes.

4. Season with salt and white pepper.
5. Plate warm brown rice, add vegetables on top and the fish.
6. Garnish with chopped coriander.

Chicken Rice Soup
4 servings
5 cups of chicken broth
2 tablespoons of cold pressed coconut oil
2 garlic cloves minced
½ kilo chicken (boneless or whatever preferred)
2 tablespoons of fish sauce
2 tablespoons of soy sauce
3 cups cooked basmati rice
1 inch piece ginger grated
½ teaspoon white pepper
1 spring onion chopped fine as garnish

1. Heat oil, add garlic and sauté. Allow to cool.
2. Heat stock in a pan, add rice and chicken and bring to a boil.
3. Add soy sauce, fish sauce, ginger and white pepper. Simmer for twenty-five seconds, until chicken is tender.
4. Transfer to serving bowl and temper with garlic warmed in oil.
5. Garnish with chopped spring onions.

Tofu Vindaloo
4 servings
500 grams tofu, cubed and cook
1½ tablespoons peeled and chopped ginger
4 garlic cloves peeled
½ teaspoon coriander pounder

½ teaspoon cardamom
½ teaspoon mustard seeds
½ teaspoon chilli powder
¼ teaspoon turmeric
½ teaspoon cumin powder
3 tablespoons olive oil
1 onion, chopped
1 large carrot cut into half moons
1 small bell pepper de-seeded and diced
400 grams tomatoes diced
¼ cup peas boiled (optional)
1 cup water
Sea or rock salt and pepper to taste

1. Blend garlic, ginger, cardamom, coriander, chilli powder, mustard seeds, cumin, cinnamon, turmeric and 1 tablespoon of ghee/oil. Blend to a paste.
2. Heat balance ghee or oil in a skillet, add onion and carrots. Cook until they turn translucent.
3. Add bell peppers, cook for about five minutes.
4. Add the paste made earlier with all spices.
5. Reduce heat and season with salt and pepper.
6. Add tomatoes and cook for a while.
7. After you see some oil leaving the mix above, add peas and water if needed and bring to a boil.
8. Cover and simmer for about 10–15 minutes more.
9. Add tofu at the end and cook for ten minutes more.
10. Serve warm.

Black Bean Cutlets with Yellow Pepper Sauce
4 servings
1½ cups cooked black beans
2 small potatoes boiled and cubed

1 cup yellow pepper sauce
½ cup onion, minced
3 tablespoon parsley, minced
½ cup carrots, grated
Sea or rock salt to taste
½ teaspoon black pepper or to taste
½ cup olive oil
Breadcrumbs (gluten-free if you are allergic to wheat)

1. Put beans and vegetables with salt and pepper in a blender.
2. Divide this mix into four cutlets, coat with breadcrumbs after shaping.
3. Coat all with breadcrumbs.
4. Put it in the fridge for thirty minutes.
5. Heat oil or ghee over medium heat. Pan fry the cutlets on both sides.
6. Eat with yellow pepper sauce.

Yellow pepper sauce
1 onion minced
3 yellow bell peppers de-seeded and chopped
Olive oil or ghee
¼ cup water

Salt and pepper
1. Heat oil or ghee over a medium flame.
2. Add onions and bell pepper. Cover and cook for ten minutes.
3. Add water and season with salt and pepper. Cook until all is soft.
4. After it cools, blend well until it is a paste.

5. Sieve through a cheesecloth or mesh.
6. Heat before serving.

Middle Eastern Lentils with Shallots and Quinoa
4 Servings
1 cup brown lentil washed after cleaning.
4 shallots (Madras onions) chopped
2 tablespoons olive oil
1 teaspoon cumin powder
1 teaspoon coriander powder
1 teaspoon red chilli powder
3 cups of water

1. Pressure cook lentils but after one whistle turn the gas off. Once the pressure comes off open the cooker and drain lentils.
2. Heat ½ the oil, add ½ the quantity of the Madras onions, cook for a while stirring frequently.
3. Add lentils to the onions, dry spices, salt and pepper.
4. Add quinoa to the lentils and water and cook through about fifteen minutes.
5. Heat the other half of the oil, add some Madras onions, cook until caramelized.
6. Place the lentil and quinoa in a bowl, garnish with caramelized onions.

Japanese Steamed Fish
500 grams salmon or a fish of your choice
4 tablespoons soy sauce
250 grams soba noodles
4 cups of vegetable stock
1-inch piece ginger grated

Fistful of broccoli cut into florets
Fistful of green beans sliced sideways
2 zucchinis sliced sideways
2 tablespoons olive oil
3 green onions sliced sideways

1. Mix together the two tablespoons of soy sauce, spoon it over the salmon and marinate in the fridge for thirty minutes.
2. Cook noodles and keep aside.
3. Bring the stock to a boil, reduce the heat; add ginger, and other vegetables, except zucchini.
4. Add the remaining soy sauce and zucchini and simmer for five minutes.
5. Heat oil in a pan, add the fish and cook for three minutes on each side.
6. Divide noodles in bowls, add stock and salmon or fish with vegetables.
7. Garnish with green onions.

Wild Mushroom Quinoa Pilaf
4 servings
1 tablespoon olive oil
2 cloves of garlic minced
1 onion diced
1 cup quinoa cooked
2 cups mushrooms (mixed mushrooms if possible)
1 tablespoon red wine vinegar
2 tablespoons parsley, chopped
Juice of 1 lemon
Sea and rock salt and black pepper to taste

1 tsp oregano
½ cup toasted walnuts or pine nuts

1. Heat olive oil in a large pan and sauté garlic and onion.
2. Add mushrooms and vinegar and season with sea salt and pepper.
3. Cook for five minutes until mushrooms are soft.
4. Mix in parsley, oregano and toasted nuts.
5. Toss in the quinoa and mix well.
6. Squeeze lime juice before serving.

Stuffed Bell Peppers with Quinoa

8 servings
4 yellow and red bell peppers
¾ cup quinoa
¼ cup black currants
2 cups water
1 cup black beans (rajma)
2 cups chopped spinach
2 cloves garlic minced
2 cups tomatoes diced
1 teaspoon coriander
2 teaspoons cumin
2 celery stalks
1 onion diced
2 tablespoons olive oil
Sea or rock salt to taste

1. Heat pan and add olive oil, onion, celery and garlic.
2. Add the dry spices and cook for five minutes until onions get soft.

3. Add tomatoes and sea salt. Cook for another five minutes.
4. Stir in black beans, black currants and quinoa with two cups of water and bring to a boil.
5. Reduce heat to low and simmer for about twenty minutes until quinoa absorbs water.
6. Pre-heat oven to 175°C.
7. Fill each bell pepper with ¼ cup quinoa.
8. Place in a baking dish and cover with foil.
9. Bake for ten minutes until you see the tops have turned brown.
10. Remove from oven and let the bell peppers sit for ten minutes before serving.

Buckwheat Noodles in Vegetable Ginger Broth

4 servings
200 grams buckwheat noodles
2 teaspoons sesame oil
2 red onions finely chopped
1-inch piece ginger
¼ cup soy sauce
4 cups vegetable stock
150 grams green beans one cut into two
2 cups mushrooms sliced thin
Handful of pak choy sliced thin
150 grams carrots cut into matchsticks
1½ cups bean sprouts washed
6 green onions cut lengthwise and long

1. Cook noodles first and rinse in cold water.
2. Cook sesame oil, onion, soy sauce and ginger. Add stock and cook for ten minutes.

3. Once it boils add carrots and mushroom. Cook for five minutes more and add bok choy and the noodles. Simmer for two minutes.
4. Finally add sprouts and green onions and serve warm.

Gado Gado
6 servings
15 leaves of spinach
2 cups cooked brown rice
½ cup of broccoli cut into florets
½ cup of red and green cabbage shredded
½ cup of carrots sliced thin
1 teaspoon garlic
1 teaspoon ginger
2 onions finely chopped
250 gms tofu
½ cup moong sprouts
Peanut sauce
1 cup organic peanut butter
1 tablespoon garlic
1 tablespoon ginger
3 tablespoons coconut sugar
1½ cups water
4 tablespoons apple cider vinegar
1 tablespoon olive oil
Sea or rock salt to taste
Blend above ingredients to make the peanut sauce and set aside.

1. Heat two tablespoons of oil in a pan. Add ginger and sauté over medium flame. Once cooked set aside to use as toppings.

2. In another pan do the same with garlic (sauté for thirty seconds only) and onions for ten minutes and set aside to use as toppings.

3. These ingredients become your toppings and should be kept aside.

4. Plate the whole dish as follows
   a. Spinach goes at the bottom (plate separately) use 4–5 leaves per plate.
   b. Add the cooked brown rice.
   c. Add the steamed vegetables: broccoli, cabbage, carrots and moong sprouts
   d. Peanut sauce goes on top of the vegetables.
   e. The toppings fried and set aside earlier go on at last.

Sweet Potato Rosti Pancakes

6 servings
4 cups grated sweet potato
½ cup onion, grated (optional)
1 teaspoon sea or rock salt
Black pepper to taste
4 tablespoons lemon juice
¼ cup flour (take more if needed to bind)
Coconut oil or whatever oil you use to pan fry

1. Combine all ingredients.
2. Heat oil in a frying pan.
3. Form pancakes with your hands.
4. Put in the frying pan.
5. Fry on both sides until light brown.

Cauliflower Marranca

6 servings
1½ cups millet (foxtail millet)
2½ cups water
2 cups onion chopped
500 grams mushrooms chopped
Pepper to taste
Sea or rock salt to taste
2 teaspoons basil
1 kilo cauliflower cut into small pieces
4 garlic cloves, minced
3 tablespoons lime juice
2 tablespoons olive oil or ghee
250 gms tofu

1. Preheat oven to 175°C.
2. Cook millet by adding water. Once done, transfer to a dish and set aside.
3. Warm oil in a pan, add onions, mushrooms, pepper and salt and sauté for 5–10 minutes.
4. Add cauliflower, basil and garlic and sauté for ten minutes more until the cauliflower is cooked; add lime juice.
5. Mix vegetables with cauliflower mix, spread on a pan and bake for fifteen minutes.
6. Remove from oven, grate tofu over dish and put in the oven again for fifteen minutes.
7. Ready to eat warm.

Sweet and Spicy Chilli

6 servings
1 onion chopped

2 garlic pods minced
2 tablespoons chilli powder
½ teaspoon cumin powder
½ teaspoon cinnamon powder
1 teaspoon sea or rock salt
3 cups tomatoes de-seeded and chopped
¾ cups tomato puree
2½ cups apple juice
2 cups vegetarian cutlet crumbled
3 cups cooked red kidney beans
½ cup toasted almonds cut lengthwise

1. Heat oil or ghee in a cooking pot using a medium flame. Add onion and garlic, cover and cook for 5–7 minutes.
2. Stir in chilli powder, cinnamon, salt and cumin powder.
3. Add tomatoes and tomato puree, kidney beans and apple juice.
4. Bring to a boil, then reduce heat.
5. Stir in the vegetable cutlet pieces.
6. Simmer for twenty minutes stirring occasionally.
7. Garnish with almonds.
8. Serve warm over rice.

Almond Bread
Makes 1 small loaf
2 cups almond flour
1 tablespoon baking powder
½ cup warm water
½ teaspoon sea or rock salt
¼ cup coconut oil
4 eggs (if non-vegetarian) or egg replacer if Vegan
¼ cup psyllium husk

1. Pre-heat oven to 175°C.
2. Mix together almond flour, psyllium husk, salt and baking powder.
3. Mix eggs or egg replacer, oil and warm water into the almond flour mix.
4. Transfer to a baking tin lined with baking paper (parchment paper).
5. Bake for 60 minutes.
6. Insert a sharp knife in the bread and if it comes out clean your bread is ready.

Almond Flour Toruntilas

Makes 6 toruntilas
1 cup almond flour
2 tablespoons psyllium husk
¼ teaspoon baking powder
½ cup warm water
1 tablespoon olive oil
Sea or rock salt to taste

1. In a mixing bowl, mix together almond flour, psyllium husk, baking powder and salt.
2. Use your hands to knead the dough. Knead for two minutes. You can add 1 tablespoon water if dough is dry. The dough should not stick to your hands.
3. Roll out dough, like you would a chapati or roti (flatbread). Here you can use a cutter to shape them perfectly or just use your rolling pin.
4. Use a pan (tava in Indian households). Add some oil cooking the toruntila like you would a chapati or a roti. Flip to other side once you feel one side is cooked well. Cook for about two minutes on each side.

5. Use a butter paper to absorb oil in between preparing each toruntila to wipe pan down.
6. Toruntilas can stay in an airtight container for up to three days in the fridge.

Flaxseed Roti (Flatbread)
½ cup flaxseed ground fine
Sea or rock salt to taste
½ cup hot water

1. Mix flaxseed powder with salt.
2. Add hot water and mix well. Set aside for ten minutes.
3. Knead well.
4. Roll after separating into balls for each roti in between butter paper sheets to prevent the roti from sticking.
5. Cook like you would cook rotis on either side.

Indian Cuisine Recipes

Sour Khatti Dal
Serves 4
1 cup split lentils with skin (green or black)
½ teaspoon chilli powder
½ teaspoon garlic minced
½ teaspoon turmeric
Rock and sea salt
Coriander leaves to garnish

1. Sort and wash dal. Soak for twenty minutes.
2. Pressure cook with 1½ cups water. After three whistles turn off and allow pressure to release.

3. Add the remaining ingredients and simmer for 7–10 minutes.
4. Garnish with coriander and serve warm.

Green Mushroom Curry

4 servings
200 grams mushrooms
¼ cup whole wheat flour for batter
1½ teaspoon garlic paste
½ teaspoon sea or rock salt
½ teaspoon pepper
½ cup water

Paste 1
¼ cup grated coconut
4 green chillies
1 onion, roughly chopped
3 flakes garlic
1 tablespoon poppy seeds (khus-khus) soaked in ¼ cup water for 10 minutes
3 tablespoons almonds
Blade of mace (javitri) crushed to get ¼ teaspoon
Seeds of 3 green cardamoms
½ teaspoon fennel seeds (saunf)

Paste 2
1½ cups coriander leaves
2 tablespoons chopped mint leaves (pudina)
1 teaspoon cumin seeds (jeera)
1 teaspoon coriander powder (dhania)
1 teaspoon coconut sugar
½ teaspoon all spice (garam masala)

¼ teaspoon mango powder (amchoor)
Sea or rock salt to taste
2 tablespoons oil or ghee

1. Wash mushrooms well. Keep mushrooms whole just trimming the stalks.
2. Mix all ingredients of the batter to make a smooth batter of coating consistency. Dip mushroom pieces in it and fry on low medium heat until light golden and cooked. Place on a paper napkin and keep aside. Alternatively use an air frier.
3. Grind all ingredients of Paste 1 to a smooth paste along with water.
4. Separately grind ingredients of Paste 2 with ½ cup water.
5. Heat 4 tablespoons of oil and cumin seeds until golden brown. Add coriander powder.
6. Add the prepared Paste 1. Sauté for 5–7 minutes stirring continuously, adding a little water if the paste sticks to the sides of the kadhai.
7. Add the prepared Paste 2. Mix and add coconut sugar, salt, garam masala and amchoor. Cook for 3–4 minutes.
8. Add two cups of water to the two pastes now mixed and simmer for five minutes.
9. At serving time, add the mushroom pieces and cook for 1–2 minutes over low heat.
10. Remove from fire. Serve hot.

Bottle Gourd (Doodhi or Lauki) with Tomatoes
4 servings
350 grams bottle gourd peeled and cut into cubes
2 onions chopped

3 tomatoes de-seeded and chopped
2 green chillies chopped
1 inch piece ginger chopped
¼ tablespoon turmeric
1 teaspoon cumin seeds (jeera)
½ teaspoon coriander powder (dhania)
1/8 teaspoon mango powder (amchoor)
½ teaspoon all spice (garam masala)
Sea or rock salt to taste
2½ tablespoons ghee or oil

1. Heat ghee in a pressure cooker and add cumin seeds. Sauté until golden.
2. Everything needs to be cooked on a medium flame and not a high flame.
3. Add onions and sauté until translucent.
4. Add ginger and green chillies. And then add turmeric.
5. After mixing well, add tomatoes.
6. Cook until all mixed well, like in India we say *bhoono* (the stage where the oil leaves the mixture) sauté well.
7. Add all the dry spices.
8. Add bottle gourd.
9. Add ½ cup of water.
10. Now pressure cook for one whistle.
11. Open cooker post pressure dropping. Simmer for five minutes.
12. Serve warm.

Turai (Ridge Gourd) Cooked with Coconut
2 servings
200 grams turai, peeled and cut into chunks
½ teaspoon red chilli powder

½ teaspoon mustard seeds
2 green chillies cut length wise into thin pieces
½ cup grated coconut
Oil or ghee as prescribed in diet

1. Warm ghee, add curry leaves and mustard seeds.
2. Add ridge gourd (turai), cover for two minutes and cook.
3. When still crunchy, add coconut.
4. Add salt and red chilli powder.
5. Garnish with coriander leaves.

Stuffed Snake Gourd (Parwals)
4 servings
200 grams snake gourd
1 onion chopped fine

Filling
1 large potato or sweet potato boiled and mashed
2 green chillies deseeded and chopped
½ inch ginger paste
¼ teaspoon turmeric powder
1 teaspoon chilli powder
Sea or rock salt to taste
½ teaspoon mango powder (amchoor)
½ teaspoon all spice, garam masala
1 tablespoon oil or ghee as prescribed
Fistful of coriander leaves chopped fine to garnish

1. Scrape the snake gourd from inside making a hollow. Split them but not fully, just from the top so you can stuff them.

2. For the filling heat the oil or ghee in a pan, add cumin seeds, ginger and green chillies and mix well. Sauté for 2–3 minutes and mix with potato or sweet potato.

3. Remove from fire and add ½ the turmeric powder, ½ chilli powder, ¼ teaspoon mango powder, ¼ teaspoon all spice and add salt to taste.

4. Stuff the hollowed-out snake gourds with the filling and pressure cook with ½ cup water and chopped coriander for one whistle.

Moong Lentil (Dal) Stuffed Green Peppers

6 servings
500 grams green peppers with head chopped off and seeds scooped out

Filling
½ cup moong lentils (dal) soaked overnight
Oil or ghee as prescribed
½ teaspoon cumin seeds
½ teaspoon coriander powder
2 tablespoon grated coconut
1 green chilly chopped
1 inch piece ginger

1. Parboil lentils.

2. Warm oil, add cumin seeds, ginger and chilli. Sauté until everything mixes well.

3. Add dry spices, coconut and salt. Cook, stirring from time to time.

4. Drain lentils after they are done. Mix with the spice mix.

5. Stuff this entire mix in each hollowed out green pepper.

6. Brush the green peppers with olive oil.
7. Preheat oven and bake at 175°C for twenty minutes.

Mung Sprouts Pav Bhaji

4 servings
4 tablespoons oil or ghee as prescribed
1½ cups tomatoes deseeded and chopped
½ cup onions grated
1 cup total (1/4 cup each) of French beans, cauliflower, red pumpkin and carrots choosing a mix of cooking styles for each vegetable
1 cup green moong sprouts steamed
½ cup potatoes, boiled
2 teaspoons chilli powder
Sea or rock salt to taste
1 tablespoon pav bhaji masala
Coriander leaves to garnish
3 tablespoons onions, chopped to garnish

1. Heat ghee or oil as prescribed.
2. Add onion and sauté until translucent.
3. Add tomatoes and dry spices. Sauté well for 5–10 minutes.
4. Add vegetables and moong sprouts.
5. Add one cup water and let it boil on a slow flame until vegetables are tender and spices have been absorbed.
6. Garnish with coriander and chopped onions.

International Cuisine Recipes

Basil Pesto

1 cup basil leaves blanched and loosely packed

1 cup walnuts or pine nuts
½ cup extra-virgin olive oil
2 teaspoons maple syrup
1 teaspoon apple cider vinegar
Some water to blend ¼ cup
Blend all ingredients together until smooth.

Falafel with Avocado and Tomato Salsa

4 servings
Falafel:
1 cup dried chickpeas and soaked overnight
1 pod garlic minced
1 teaspoon coriander powder
1 teaspoon cumin powder
½ teaspoon chilli powder
3 tablespoons each of coriander and parsley
2 green onions chopped
4 tablespoons cold-pressed sesame oil
Sea and rock salt to taste

Salsa:
1 avocado scooped and chopped
3 tomatoes, deseeded and chopped
1 onion chopped
2 red chilies deseeded and chopped
2 tablespoons coriander leaves
Juice of 1 lime
3 tablespoons of extra-virgin olive oil
Sea or rock salt to taste
Chop and mix all ingredients of salsa.

1. Drain and dry chickpeas with a napkin.
2. Use a food processor and add chickpeas and dry spices including garlic.
3. Set aside in a bowl in the fridge for 15–20 minutes.
4. Add parsley, coriander and green onions.
5. Spoon out small round balls and shape into round patties ½-inch thick.
6. Pan fry and cook falafel on each side until brown.
7. Enjoy the falafel with salsa.

Sweet Potato and Broccoli Salad
6 servings
Salad:
500 gm broccoli cut into florets and steamed
3 medium sized sweet potatoes sliced and steamed or boiled

Marinade:
½ cup olive or avocado oil
3 tablespoons lemon juice
2 tablespoons red wine vinegar
2 garlic pods minced
Sea or rock salt to taste
1 tablespoon ground mustard
¼ teaspoon stevia
Freshly ground black pepper

1. Combine the marinade in a bowl.
2. Add sweet potato slices to marinade and chill for 2–4 hours.
3. Before serving mix in broccoli.

Caramelized Onion Sauce with Quinoa Pasta

6 servings
¼ cup olive oil
5 large onions sliced thin
1 bunch any leafy green minced
½ cup white wine
Sea and rock salt to taste
450 grams quinoa pasta or pasta of-choice
Vegans add almond feta
Non-Vegans add choice of meats and feta cheese
Garnish with coriander leaves

1. Heat oil in a deep pan and add onions. Sauté for 10–15 minutes until translucent.
2. Add salt and cook for at least ten minutes.
3. Add white wine and let it simmer for twenty minutes. Set aside.
4. Take the sauce back to the flame, add greens or vegetables of choice. Sauté for a few minutes.
5. Mix in feta cheese. Cook on a low flame.
6. Add sauce to cooked pasta and garnish with coriander leaves.

18

The Hormone-Transformation Exercise Plan

'It's not about perfect. It's about effort. And when you bring that effort every single day, that's where transformation happens.'

—Jillian Michaels

One of the best things I did for myself was to get certified in the Louise Solomon Yogalates method. I did the programme in Byron Bay, Australia, in 2006, when I spent a year there as a resident Yogalates student. I was an athlete in school, ran long distance and played hockey, representing my school, AF Petit High School, which made sure we had plenty to do if we were inclined towards sports. I suffered with back pain and my family put it down to faulty genes that I inherited from my father. In retrospect, it was my weak digestive system, which I have talked about extensively in my book The Detox Diet. *Due to my back problems, I enrolled in a yoga class with a very reputed teacher from the Santacruz Yoga Institute, Bubbles Sahani. While still a student, I pushed off to the US for my master's degree. I did a lot of aerobics, ran 8 kms on the beach every day, did weight training and then yoga. I must admit that exercise is one aspect of my life that has kept me sane, happy and strong. In school, we have no desire to look slim; but simply participate in sports event, but once out of school, weight loss becomes the goal for many women. At St Xavier's, the college I went to, we had an abundance of cute guys and parties galore, so looking slim was my goal, like any sixteen-year-old. As time went on, I lost all my puppy fat and staying fit was just hardwired into my DNA. My father was a swimmer (100 laps in an Olympic-size pool every other day) and a walker (8–10 kms a day). He was also the one who brought every book on fitness and nutrition into our house, exposing me to the disciplines of health and importance of diet and lifestyle at an early age.*

I really started focusing on my core and pelvic health when I came down with a slip disk at the age of thirty and was bedridden for three months. With nothing to do, I decided to get Louise Solomon's DVDs and practised her approach in bed. Her approach is a combination of yoga and Pilates and every day I got better and better. Pilates focuses on the core, the girdle of muscle that surrounds the midsection of the body.

While many people use the term abs interchangeably with the core, this is incorrect. Abs concerns the rectus abdominus muscles, the paired muscles that run down the front of the abdominal wall. These make up the six-pack that a John Abraham or Shah Rukh Khan show off in films. The core, on the other hand, is the bridge between the upper torso and the legs. It is the source of stability during daily- and exercise-related activities and protects your internal organs and stabilizes the spine. A weak core will make your back vulnerable to injury. The core includes the rectus abdominus, the internal and external oblique muscles, transverse abdominus muscle, the pelvic floor and the paraspinal muscles, erector spinae, multifidus and psoas.

Shonali Sabherwal

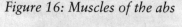

Figure 16: Muscles of the abs

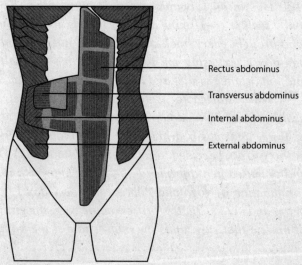

Rectus abdominus

Transversus abdominus

Internal abdominus

External abdominus

The Physics of the Pelvic Girdle

The foundation of all support of the structures in the abdomen and pelvis is the pelvic floor or the pelvic girdle, also called the pelvic diaphragm or the pelvic platform. As the names suggest, the pelvic floor is made up of the group of muscles and ligaments that form a hammock-like sling that runs run from front to back, attached to the pubic bone at one end and the tail bone at the other. It can be activated by simply imagining that you want to stop your pee and clenching the muscles that do that for you. Women do not pay enough attention to this area of their body. While most yoga and Pilates classes focus on the core, women still need an education about and awareness of this part of their anatomy.

The pelvic floor and the core need constant exercise. This was the biggest benefit of Shonali's Yogalates training and also why she recovered completely from her slip disk. Weak pelvic floor muscles are further weakened by the pressure put on them by the upper body during any form of exercise like running, strength training, functional training, dance classes, aerobics and all physical activity involving movement. In the long run, signs of a weak pelvic floor involve leaking of urine when coughing, sneezing or running, prolapsed uterus, urethrocele (prolapse of the female urethra into the vagina), reduced vaginal sensation and a feeling of heaviness in the vagina. Issues that impair pelvic health in the long run include pregnancy, vaginal birth, obesity, chronic constipation, lower estrogen levels post-menopause or even a chronic cough that lasts a long time.

The Perimenopausal Woman and Pelvic Power

When Shonali's teacher, Louise Solomon, mentioned the pelvic area, she always said,

> . . . let's bring our attention to the pelvic area which not only houses the reproductive organs, but is also the *seat* of sexual sensitivity.[*]

A strong pelvic girdle will not only help you in the bedroom (by this I mean, have great sex), it houses much more. It is the core of emotional intuition and is the centre for all your creative energy.

Understanding Your Core

Every Yogalates movement revolves around the core of your body, that is the skeleton, spine and the pelvis. The core provides you with stability, a foundation, a base from which everything (movement-wise) needs to be layered to prevent injury.

The spine is literally the backbone of everything in your life. The author, Louise Hay,[†] says that the spine shows 'flexibility and support' in your life. Any issues with the spine will show as a rage towards life, inflamed thinking and the inability to flow with life. Fear and trying to hold on to old ideas will show the person as not trusting life, lacking in integrity and having no courage of conviction. While you must question all of these issues if you are dealing with an

---

[*] Solomon, Louise *Yogalates: Total Body Toner*, Virgin Books, 2003, p. 22.

[†] Hay, Louise L., *You Can Heal Your Life*, Full Circle, 1984, p. 200.

issue concerning the spine, on a physical level we can do a lot in this section to set things right.

The spine has twenty-four vertebrae which articulate with one another to create a delicately balanced tower of great structural integrity and capable of movement in all directions. A healthy spin forms three natural curves which she calls the neutral spine concept. The 'lumbar spine' with five vertebrae starting at the bottom (tailbone) forms the first natural curve of the spine and is the lower back. The 'thoracic spine' consists of the next twelve vertebrae curves towards the back of the body and this forms the second natural curve and is the mid-back. The 'cervical spine' with seven vertebrae forms the third natural curve that supports the weight of the head and is the neck. The spine contains, protects and carries the spinal cord which is the part of the central nervous system (CNS) that runs from the base of the skull down to the beginning of the lumbar curve. All the three sections of the spine, lumbar, thoracic and cervical, work synergistically to help with movement.

When Shonali's slip disk happened, she lost sensation in the toes of her right foot because some nerves were being pinched along her lumbar spine. The spine houses many nerves that exit through openings in the vertebrae. The CNS is constantly sending messages from the brain in the skull down to the back of the pelvis and to the muscles for control of movement with the receptors in your muscles sending back messages regarding movement and balance to the brain. The Yogalates method impacts not just the pelvis, but also the spine and all the major organs in the body, with the 'core' remaining the focal centre of everything.

The core is essentially the centre of the body and is key in terms of performance, functionality and longevity. The core is called upon when firing each and every muscle in your body. For example, when you squat, your core is engaged to maintain the integrity of the movement, when pressing dumbbells overhead the core keeps the body straight as opposed to curved.

Core exercises enable the skeleton, muscles and joints to work together properly, while offering a combination of strengthening, elasticity, balance, realignment and fat loss—things that nutrition alone would not achieve. Core exercises are a group of exercises, movements and positions that target the core directly. Core stability on the other hand are those movements and physical positions that help build a strong core that is then ready to do whatever you ask of it.

The Hormone-Transformation Exercise Plan for Pelvic Health

Coming from the Solomon Yogalates tradition that has given her core health, Shonali has outlined a Yogalates exercise plan that is easy, can be practised at home or when you travel and it scores over just doing a regular yoga practice because it focuses on the core through each exercise. This plan offers great advantage to women going through perimenopause or menopause and additional exercise plans are suggested to strengthen bones and muscles. Visit soulfoodshonali.com for details of exercises referred to in the transformation exercise plan.

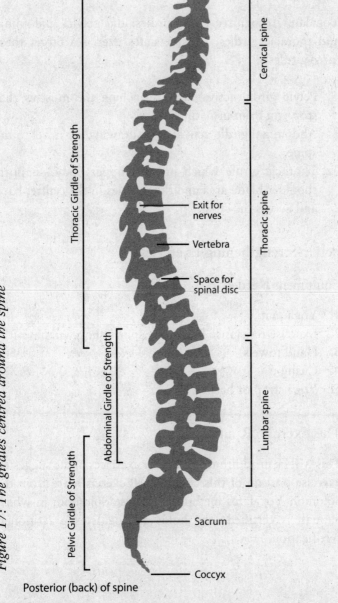

Figure 17: The girdles centred around the spine

Anterior (front) of spine

Cervical spine

Thoracic spine

Lumbar spine

Thoracic Girdle of Strength

Abdominal Girdle of Strength

Pelvic Girdle of Strength

Exit for nerves

Vertebra

Space for spinal disc

Sacrum

Coccyx

Posterior (back) of spine

Yogalates and the Three Girdles

Yogalates recognizes three girdles: the pelvic, abdominal and thoracic girdles. All Yogalates exercises target these three girdles.

A. Pelvic girdle activated by clenching the muscles that stop you from urinating.
B. Abdominal girdle activated by drawing the navel to the spine.
C. Thoracic girdle which protects upper body, supports shoulder blade area and the muscles in the centre, back and across the chest.

Pelvic-Strengthening Exercises

Equipment Needed

1. Yoga mat
2. Exercise resistance band (any sports shop will have it)
3. Hand towels
4. Cushion
5. Yoga strap or belt

The Exercise Routine

This will be in addition to all other exercises in the suggested exercise portion of this chapter. All exercises are from the Solomon Yogalates method by Louise Solomon, in which Shonali is certified—she holds a 'Yogalates practitioner' certification.

Exercise 1

To check for the position from which all movement will be initiated, start by lying supine and flat on a yoga mat. Your legs and feet are relaxed, and arms are at the side of the body (like in Shavasana). Keep your arms at a 45° angle from your body (thighs) and check for the following:

1. Hip bones are parallel.
2. Neck and chin are pointing towards the ceiling.
3. You can place a rolled hand towel under your head.
4. Slide a pillow or bolster under your knees.
5. Plug into your breath.
6. Inhale and when you exhale feel the body sink deeper into the mat.
7. Feel the back of your pelvis indent itself on your mat.
8. Now walk up the spine to your lumbar spine which arches off the floor.
9. Walk further up and feel the thoracic spine indent back on the floor.
10. Walk further up and feel the cervical spine arching off the floor.

Remember this as the position of your body's natural alignment.

Exercise 2: Supine Rest Position

1. Place your palms on your hip bones.
2. Inhale and as you exhale feel the navel drop towards the spine and slide your left foot up and then the right foot up, keeping your knees bent.

3. This position puts the spine in an anti-gravity position.
4. This is a great position to rest and take a break from your daily activities.
5. Initiate all movement in other exercises from this supine rest position.

Exercise 3: Breathing

Part 1 Thoracic Girdle Activation

Yogalates practice always emphasizes breathing as the breath is the bridge between the mind and the body. Breathe in and out through the nose and use the lateral thoracic breathing system. The breathing technique used is called lateral thoracic breathing.

1. Lie in supine rest position described in Exercise 2.
2. Take normal natural breaths.
3. As you inhale feel the rib cage and abdomen rise and as you exhale feel them sink gently.
4. Draw the navel towards the back of the spine with an activation of the abdominal girdle.
5. Take a few breaths in this position to get in tune with your abdominal girdle.
6. On your next exhale put a little more weight into the abdomen and sink the navel to the spine feeling the weight in this area.
7. When you repeat this again keep the navel retracted and now inhale and you will notice the breath will jump into your chest or ribcage, which is a sign of the activation of the thoracic breathing system.

8. Place your hand on either side of the rib cage with fingertips touching and repeat this breathing. When you hold the navel to the spine and breathe into the ribcage you will feel the fingertips separating.

9. Exhale and feel the ribcage compress and inhale feel the fingertips separate.

Part 2 Pelvic Girdle Activation

1. Place both hands on your hip bone and put your fingertips on the pubic bone the bony part of your pelvis.

2. Inhale ballooning the belly out and exhale to drop navel to the spine. Now draw in the pelvic muscles as if to prevent yourself from urinating.

3. Repeat this again to experience how to engage the pelvic girdle

Exercise 4: Cushion or Block Squeeze

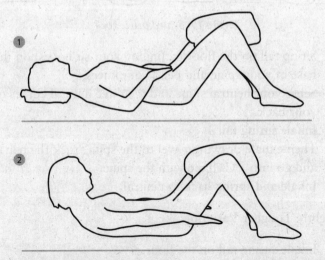

Figure 18: Cushion or block squeeze to activate the pelvic girdle

1. Lie down in supine rest position.
2. Stick a cushion or a yoga block between the knees.
3. Place both palms on your hip bone.
4. Inhale ballooning the belly out and exhale, sinking the abdomen to the spine.
5. As you do this squeeze the cushion between your knees.
6. Repeat this exercise 5 times.

Exercise 5: Seated Pelvic Rock

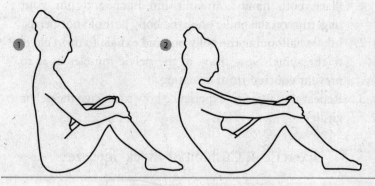

Figure 19: Seated pelvic rock

1. Sit up tall on the floor (sitting on your sit bones) on the base of your spine and bend your knees.
2. Sense your neutral spine and the three natural curves of your back.
3. Inhale sitting tall.
4. Then exhale drawing navel to the spine, tuck the pelvis and go into a C-shape with the spine.
5. Inhale and spring back to neutral.

Slightly Tougher Variation

1. Inhale sitting tall on the floor.
2. As you exhale, lean back 6 inches, then hold.

3. Drawing the navel to the spine, inhale.
4. Exhale go down 6 inches more hold and inhale.
5. Exhale 6 inches leaning back even further, then hold.
6. Exhale coming back to neutral spine, sitting tall.

Exercise 6: Abdominal Roll-Down Series

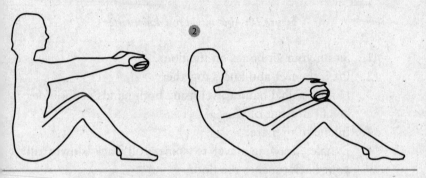

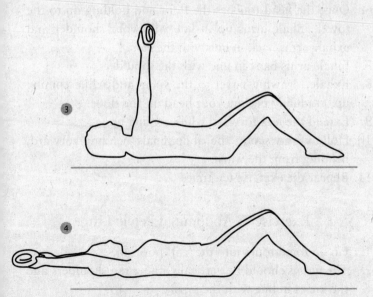

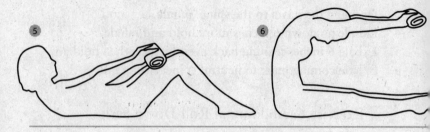

Figure 20: Abdominal roll down series

1. Sit on your sit bones on the floor.
2. Press the feet and knees together.
3. Hold a rolled hand towel using both hands at shoulder height in front of you.
4. Inhale to prepare.
5. Exhale, drawing navel to spine, roll back slowly till your back touches the floor.
6. Once the head touches the floor and holding on to the towel, inhale arms up in line with your shoulder and exhale arms back in line with the ears.
7. Inhale arms back in line with the shoulders.
8. Exhale, drawing navel to the spine and while coming up, gradually peeling your head off the floor.
9. Extend the legs forward while coming up.
10. Hollow and scoop the abdominals bending forward, bending from the waist.
11. Repeat the exercise ten times

Exercise 7: Abdominal Pelvic Lift

1. Go on to all fours into the 'cat' position.
2. The wrists should be vertically under the shoulders and the knees in line with the hips.

3. Spread the palms on the floor, pointing middle finger forwards.
4. Find neutral spine, extend the spine through the crown of your head to the tail bone.
5. Look down on to the floor.
6. Slide shoulders back into the thoracic upper part behind the shoulder blades.
7. Now without moving the spine inhale to prepare.
8. Exhale and draw the navel to the spine with three tiny contractions like you are pulsing the breath.
9. Sense the abdominals go hollow towards the spine.
10. Inhale and release the abdominals towards the floor.
11. Repeat the exercise five times

Exercise 8: Wall Sits

1. Stand against a wall.
2. Lean against it and take your feet forward.
3. Slide down the wall into a seated position, pretending you are sitting on a chair.
4. The lower back, mid-back and upper back should rest against the wall.
5. Raise your arms forward shoulder length, they should be parallel to the floor.
6. Hold this pose for sixty seconds then come up.
7. Complete five repetitions of the exercise.

Exercise 9: Bridge Pose

1. Lie on your back in supine rest position with feet closer to the butt.

2. Arms should be extended to either side, palms face down and flat on the floor.
3. Inhale then exhale retracting the navel to the spine and lift your butt off the floor.
4. Push through your heels as you lift the pelvis until your torso is aligned with your thighs and hold for thirty seconds.
5. Push through your heels and not your toes.
6. Inhale and exhale, pulling navel to the spine, coming back to the floor and layering one vertebra at a time on the floor.

Exercise 10: The Plank

1. Start by coming on your tip toes with hands palms down.
2. The hands should be parallel to one another and in push-up position.
3. Keep chest uplifted, knees off the floor and extend legs.
4. Remain there for thirty seconds and gradually build this up to one minute.
5. Keep chest and abdominal muscles active. Engage the core by pulling navel to spine.

Exercise 11: The Clam

1. Start by lying on one side. Hold the waist up off the floor through the activation of abdominal and pelvic girdle.
2. Place hand in front of the chest for extra stability.
3. Inhale, hunch the upper shoulders towards the ear, shortening the neck muscles.

4. Exhale, slide the shoulder away from the ears, lengthening the neck, keep this distance through the exercise.
5. Inhale.
6. Exhale, draw navel to the spine, keep feet together open knee towards the ceiling and squeeze your butt. There should be no movement in the pelvis.
7. Inhale and release back down, joining knees back again.
8. Repeat about twenty times on each side.

Exercise 12: Jellyfish

1. Lying in supine rest, draw one knee at a time into the chest. Knees should be wide, flatten the lower back and pelvis on the floor.
2. Opening hips, hold each knee from the top.
3. Inhale.
4. Exhale, navel to spine and take both knees in a clockwise motion ten times and repeat anti-clockwise ten times.

While the exercise routines suggested above are fabulous for a strong 'core' and pelvic health, there are many other types of exercises you can engage in. Let's have a look at each, so you have options to choose from.

Yoga for Perimenopausal Health

India has an amazing tradition of yoga, a tradition that has an amazing way to free up your body, bring it into alignment, iron out muscular imbalances and improve strength and physical weaknesses. You can enhance flexibility by using the breathing techniques of pranayama to relax in all those anxious moments you go through and create balance in your life. Shonali's understanding from her personal experience with yoga is that not every style works for everyone, so make sure you go with a teacher who fits with you. When she realized that *ashtanga yoga* was not for her, she started with *hatha yoga*, graduated to *Yogalates* (combination of the T.K.V. Desikachar style of yoga with Pilates) and also does some *Iyengar yoga*. With yoga, consistent practice is very important. It requires discipline and commitment, but it's the best gift you will give to yourself.

Yoga can alleviate menopausal symptoms such as hot flashes, mood swings, weak bones, depression and insomnia that accompany menopause. The deep breathing and relaxation prescribed in pranayama is beneficial for blood circulation, maintaining muscle tone and flexibility and increasing the levels of mood-regulating chemicals in the brain. Yoga massages the internal organs, nourishing them with increased blood circulation, as well as toning the interior and exterior muscles. Yoga also provides effective, weight-bearing exercises that strengthen bones. It lowers cholesterol and improves heart efficiency.

Why Are Inversions (Asanas That Lift the Feet above the Head) Good for You?

Here's a true story featuring Dr Nozer and me. I'm trying to break the monotony of your reading this book, and a funny story is a funny story. I am going to call it: 'The story of how inversions and macrobiotics helped me get rid of some unidentified stuff down there'—yes, by 'down there' I mean in my vagina.

I was studying in Australia to be a yoga Pilates instructor. The core is the major focus of anything we do in this practice, so there was a lot of yoga practice (four hours a day) and lots of core work. I was dealing with my recurring candida issues and addressing it with my diet as I was simultaneously pursuing my Macrobiotics Nutritionist and Chef course in America. I was in between my levels so I was my own guinea pig. I was determined to get rid of my candida with the macrobiotic approach, so I was doing sitz baths (with hips immersed in hot water) the water boiled with radish (mooli) leaves. In macrobiotics, this gets rid of unwanted fat and mucus accumulation in the area. I dried my radish leaves religiously and my landlady, who is one of my dear friends now, would make fun of me as the kitchen would stink of dried radish.

One day, I felt something sticking out of my vaginal opening. I used a mirror to see what was going on and saw a bulge. I was surprised. I had seen my mother's prolapsed uterus, although hers was worse and she lived with it for many years. I was to return to India for a break before going off to America, so I scheduled an appointment with Dr Nozer.

As I lay on his table, deeply worried, he walked in, calm, composed and smiling as always. Just one glimpse of him and you would melt into the examination table.

Oh, I forgot to mention this . . . I went to another gynaecologist first because Dr Nozer had been out of town. That gynaecologist had a more radical approach and announced that it was a urethrocele (a prolapse of the female urethra into the vagina) which happens when the pelvic floor gets weak. She wanted to fix it with a surgical procedure. However, in my heart I knew that this couldn't possibly be true because my core had never felt better, and I knew my pelvic floor was strong. So, I decided to wait and then, when Dr Nozer came back, went straight to see him.

So, this is him, examining me. He says that he has no answer for what this might be, but that my pelvic floor was probably too strong and that, with all the exercises I had been doing, one of the vaginal folds had decided to say hello. He asked me to just continue to do what I had been doing and to see him when I got back to India (this time, I was going to be gone for a good nine months).

Mind you, this thing never bothered me; it wasn't that large; it jutted out maybe half an inch and I wasn't sexually active at the time as I had no time—I was too busy studying between the two countries, America and Australia, and had no time to meet boys. Back in Australia, I just carried on with my diet, the sitz baths, my Yogalates practice and here, might I add, a lot of inversions (inverted poses).

Back in India, after nine months, I went and met Dr Nozer. I had stopped paying attention to my vagina, but the thought remained at the back of my

> *mind that I needed to get re-examined. Same story, Dr Nozer glides in, asks me how I was doing and then looks up at me, saying, 'it's gone'.*
>
> *I was surprised. He repeated, yes, it was no longer there. Perhaps with all the pelvic floor exercises and the natural remedies, things just got better 'down there'.*
>
> *Shonali Sabherwal*

Coming to the moral of the story: yoga asana 'inversions' are the best for your hormonal circuitry, so do use all the inversions listed in the chart put together on poses with their benefits. Dr Karen Koffler, former director of Integrative Medicine at Evanston Northwestern Hospital, explains the benefits of inversions for the brain:

Inverted positions that are assumed in yoga alter the blood flow (including lymphatic drainage) and flow of cerebral spinal fluid (CSF). If there is increased blood flow to the area, there will be increased bioavailability of oxygen and glucose—the two most important metabolic substrates for the brain. It follows then that cells bathed in a solution that is rich in factors required for the creation of neurotransmitters (like norepinephrine, dopamine, and serotonin) will be better able to produce these chemicals.[*]

Inversions positively impact the endocrine system, which is a network of glands (an organ that makes and puts out hormones) in your body that produce the hormones that help

---

[*] Ghin, Stacy Lee, 'Why Inversions are Good for Your Mind', *wanderlust. com*.

cells communicate with each other. They are responsible for every cell, organ and function in your body. Many glands make up the endocrine system: the hypothalamus, pituitary and pineal gland are a part of your brain; the thymus is between your lungs; the adrenals are on top of your kidneys; and the pancreas is behind the stomach. Your ovaries are in your pelvic region. Endocrine system disorders range from hypothyroid, hyperthyroid, polycystic ovaries, hypopituitarism, Cushing's disease, adrenal insufficiency and acromegaly.

So, how is it possible that inversions will affect the endocrine system? During an inversion, when the endocrine glands are saturated in blood, they absorb nutrients from it and then secrete hormones into it. When you assist the endocrine system with gravity, inversion causes venous blood from the lower extremities to drain towards the heart. The increased blood flow stimulates a healthier exchange of nutrients and also flushes out wastes from the endocrine glands. This will aid circulation of hormones in the vascular system more efficiently to other parts of the body.

Outlined here are the various inversions. The easiest one you can do on your own is Downward-Facing Dog (*adho mukha svanasana*). Do ask your yoga teacher about the other inversions highlighted and do get going with them if possible. While you can keep up with a regular yoga practice, stressing on the pelvic floor, inversions and restorative yoga is a must. A lot of the women understand yoga but do not understand the immense benefits of 'inversions' and the impact they have on the endocrine system and hormones.

Core Lengthening, Inversions and Restorative Poses

Core lengthening	Benefits
	Teaches spinal alignment
	Establishes optimum movement position.
	Establishes neutral spine
	Stabilizes muscles of the torso
	Stabilizes thoracic breath
	Holds the muscles that attach to pelvis in balance
	Strengthens pelvic girdle
	Aids shoulder plus scapular stabilization
	Establishes a point of return after each pose
	Develops stability
	Corrects posture
	Cultivates alertness (*sthira*)
	Lifts abdomen and tones it
Yoga poses that achieve core-lengthening	Upwards hand pose (*urdhva hastasana*)
	Half dog or right-angle pose (*ardha svanasana*)
	Full body-stretch, lying down (*tadasana*)
Hip and butt poses	Strengthens buttocks, thighs and hip
	Builds flexibility in the hips and pelvic area
	Stretches quadriceps
	The Bridge (*setu bandhasana*)
	Develops tremendous strength and spine flexibility
	Strengthens buttocks, shoulder, back, arms and feet
	Stretches pelvic region, abdominals and quadriceps
	Exhilarating, energizing, calming and tension-relieving
	Keeps body alert and mind clear

	The Clam All muscles of buttock toned Firms inner and outer thighs Stabilizes pelvis and hips **The Jellyfish** Hips get more circulation Increases hip flexibility Stabilizes pelvis and hips arms inner thighs
Inversions	**Overall benefits** Revitalizes the whole system Floods the brain with nutrients Activates pineal and pituitary glands (endocrine system) Improves circulation, venous return and lymph drainage Relieves fatigue in legs and feet Stimulates intestinal sluggishness Aids digestion and sleep Increases core strength Gives a new perspective to life and helps you relax
Inversions in yoga	Headstand (*shirshasana*) Shoulder stand (*sarvangasana*) Standing forward fold (*uttanasana*) Wide-legged forward bend (*prasarita padottanasana*) Downward dog (*adho mukha svanasana*) Legs up the wall (*viparita karani*)

Restorative yoga	Revitalizes the whole system
	Cleansing and nourishing at deeper levels
	Tremendous systemic harmonization and health
	Energizing, calming and soothing
	Clears the mind
	All parts of the body; skin, muscles and nerves relax
	Relieves strain and fatigue
	Conducive to meditation
	Mood stabilizer
	Reduces fatigue, adrenal stress and immune depletion
Yoga poses	Corpse pose (shavasana)
	Reclining kneeling pose (*supta virasana*)
	Child pose (*balasana*)
	Legs up the wall (viparita karani)
	Reclining twist with bolster
	Supported seated angle pose
	Crocodile pose (*makrasana*)

Women's Health Issues during Menopause and Yoga Poses to Achieve Balance

Women's health	Yoga poses to handle them
Breast health	Child pose (balasana)
	Seated spinal twist (marichyasana)
	Warrior pose 2 (virabhadrasana 2)
	Backbend (chakrasana)
	Reclining supine twist (supta matseyendra)
	Fish pose (matsyasana)
	Staff pose (dandasana)

Constipation Digestion	Bow (dhanurasana) Fish (matsyasana) Plough (halasana) Twists (marichiasana, bharadvajasana, trikonasana, supta matsyendrasana) Revolved-triangle pose (trikonasana revolved) Cat-cow pose (marjaryasana-bitilasana) Downward-facing dog (adho mukha svanasana) Triangle pose (trikonasana) Extended puppy pose (uttnasana shishosana) Bridge pose (setu bandha sarvangasana) Half-gas pose (ardha pawamuktasana)
Depression Mood swings	Alternate nostril breathing (anulom-vilom) Belly breath, complete breath, bee-breathing technique (bhramari) Corpse pose (shavasana) Mountain pose (tadasana) Shoulder stand (sarvangasana) Sun salutation (surya namaskar) Yoga mudra
Endometriosis	All pelvic poses highlighted in previous chart Seated wide angle pose (upavistha konasana) Camel pose (ustrasana) Reclining-cobbler's pose (supta baddha konasana) Lying-down hero pose (supta virasana) Shoulder stand (sarvangasana) Corpse (shavasana)

Fibroids	Garland pose (malasana)
	Standing forward fold (padahastasana)
	Wind-removing pose (pavanmuktasana)
	Half-fish pose (ardha matsyendra asana)
	Cobbler's pose (baddha konasana)
	Sage pose (bharadvajasana)
	Seated forward bend (paschim utthasasana)
Hair Issues	Scalp stimulator modified head stand (sirsasana)
	Cobra pose (bhujangasana)
	Locust pose (salabhasana)
	Mountain pose (tadasana)
Hot flashes **Hot flushes**	Lying-down cobbler's pose (supta baddha konasana)
	Half-plough pose (*ardha halasana*)
	All restorative poses in the previous chart
	Seated forward bend (paschim utthasasana)
	Standing forward fold (*padahastasana*)
Hysterectomy	Hero pose (*virasana*)
	Lying-down-hero pose (supta virasana)
	Legs-up-the-wall pose (viparita karani)
	Cat pose (marjaryasana)
	Cobra pose (bhujangasana)
	Warrior pose 1 (virabhadrasana 1)
	Half lord-of-the-fishes pose (ardha matsyendrasana)
	All the poses highlighted in the restorative section of the previous chart

Incontinence	Ashwini mudra acts as a perineal seal plus tightens the pelvic diaphragm and anal sphincter All exercises highlighted in the previous chart for strengthening the pelvic floor engaging the *mulabandha* (root lock in the yogic system) or pelvic platform in Pilates (Kegels) Chair pose (utkatasana) Cobbler's pose (baddha konasana) Upward salute (urdhva hastasana)
Sleeplessness Insomnia	Inversions (uttanasana, adho mukha svanasana, sirsasana, prasarita paddotasana) Shoulder stand (sarvangasana)
Lack of energy	All inversions as specified in previous chart Corpse (shavasana) Yoga mudra Easy pose with an arch (sukhasana) Upward Salute (urdhva hastasana) Low cobra pose (ardha bhujhangasana) Locust pose (salabhasana) Full cobra pose (bhujangasana) Upward-facing-dog pose (urdhva mukha svanasana) Low lunge with an arch (*anjaneyasana*) Upward salute with an arch (urdhva hastasana) Fish pose (matsyasana) Bow pose (dhanurasana) Camel pose (ustrasana)

Menstrual regulation	Bow pose (dhanurasana) Cobra pose (bhujangasana) Fish pose (matsyasana) Locust pose (salabhasana) Plough pose (halasana) Shoulder stand (sarvangasana)
Memory Alzheimer's	All Inversions Downward-facing dog (adho mukga svanasana) Corpse pose (shavasana)
Migraines	Lying-down-cobbler's pose (supta baddha konasana) All inversions Corpse pose (shavasana) Standing forward fold (hastpadasana) Bridge pose (setu bhandhasana) Cat pose (marjariasana) Child pose (balasana) Seated forward bend (paschimottanasana) Lotus pose (padmasana)
Osteoporosis	Mountain pose (tadasana) Sun salutation (surya namaskar) All weight-bearing poses
PCOS	All poses listed in the weight-gain section of this chart
Ovaries	Supine-cobbler's pose (supta baddha konasana) Child pose (balasana) Sage pose (bharadvajasana) Plough pose (halasana) Breathing (*kapalbhati*) *Yoni* mudra Bow pose (dhanurasana)

Reproductive Organs	Bow pose (dhanurasana) Cobra pose (bhujangasana) Locust pose (salabhasana) See all pelvis exercises suggested in the previous chart
Sex	Complete breath Plough pose (halasana) Shoulder stand (sarvangasana)
Skin Anti-wrinkle	Lion pose (*simhasana*) Modified head stand (sirsasana) Sun Salutation (surya namaskar) Shoulder stand (sarvangasana)
Weight	Bow pose (dhanurasana) Cobra pose (bhujangasana) Locust pose (salabhasana) Shoulder stand (sarvangasana) Sun salutation (surya namaskar) Shoulder stand (sarvangasana) Warrior 1,2,3, (virabhadrasana 1,2,3) Triangle pose (trikonasana) Boat pose (*navasana*) Four-limbed staff pose (plank) Seated forward bend (paschimottanasana) Upward-facing dog (urdhva mukha svanasana)

Cardio for Perimenopausal Health

Building in some cardio to combat the fat gain during this time is necessary, but also look at your cardio as a means to keep up your cardiovascular health. Do not indulge in very intense workouts, but instead use this time to get started with some sort of strength training after you finish the first two phases of the diet plan. During the hormone-transformation-diet plan, I want to prepare you for a suitable strengthening technique which you will use after you get on to a maintenance plan. So, whether you walk, skip, use the treadmill, run on the beach, in the garden or on the roads (not ideal for the back), engage in functional training, swimming or biking; engage in the exercise for thirty minutes at least four times a week.

Make it your goal to have cardio in your life always, every day or at least four times a week. Cardio makes your lungs work harder, your heart work better. It helps burn all that belly fat, and fat around your hips and thighs. Do not over-exercise as this will lead to stress, higher cortisol levels, increased free radical damage, all inducing poor recovery post-exercise as well as loss of muscle and as a consequence you will lose the benefits of working out. To give you a perfect balance of yin and yang in terms of activity

- Take breaks between intense training days.
- Set realistic and achievable goals.
- Team up with your spouse or friends to help you stay motivated.
- Engage in one day of functional training (which is intense) and do yoga or swimming on the other days.

Here is a list of activities which you can engage in at home for a cardio, without equipment. As you know, walking, jogging (if your knees and back permit), cycling, aerobics, a dance class, any form of functional training and anything that ups your heart rate, all are a part of the cardio activity you can do.

- Climbing stairs
- Jumping Jacks
- Up-and-down a step or a stool

- Knee kicks
- Boxing
- Burpees
- Skipping

Massage for Perimenopausal Health

When women think of massages, they think of them as an indulgence, but if you change the lens through which you look at massages, as being therapeutic, they take on a whole new meaning.

Massages are a gift you can give yourself during this time. They are a powerful tool that will help you achieve a state of wellbeing both physically and mentally. Any kind of massage can help during this time. While deep tissue massages are popular, there are several types of massages that you can choose from based on your preference.

They have the following benefits:

- Help the lymphatic system discharge toxins
- Reduced stress and anxiety
- Increased relaxation response
- Help with soreness after exercise
- Increased circulation of blood flow to all organs
- Lowered heart rate
- Help you sleep better
- Improved immune function
- Normalize muscles, connective tissue, tendons and ligaments

You can choose how often you'd like to take a massage. Usually taking a massage twice a week can complement your exercise schedule. Make sure you do not suffer from injuries, or do not have your period when you take a massage. If you suffer from chronic inflammation, especially related to the bones or ligaments, talk to your doctor about massages.

Meditate for Perimenopausal Health

My relationship with vipassana meditation is presented in greater detail in my earlier book, but here is a smattering of that story.

As a child, I was spiritually inclined, although at the time I didn't know that I had chosen a life to learn my lessons (reap my karma) and work towards the negativity that I had within me. We all have some traces of negativity and life's situations push these karmas to the surface and force us to examine them. Whether we choose to learn from them or not is entirely our call. I now realize that I was born to learn from them. I can safely say that the technique of vipassana changed me as a person. Now that I have been practising it for twenty-five years, I believe it is the most powerful tool you can use to keep you calm, centred and truly objective about people, situations and events that don't serve you. For those of you going through this time of perimenopause, it is the best tool to re-balance your hormones.

I have practised my meditation diligently and it is now such an intrinsic part of my life that I take for granted. Sitting for one, sometimes two, hours of meditation is something I have done religiously for

> twenty-five years. Attending courses at the Vipassana International Academy is something that is just hardwired into my system. I have over the last twenty-five years, done twenty-four courses, and this includes twenty- and thirty-day courses. I say this with no ego, and I don't think twice when I enrol or how my work and my business will manage without me. I just go as the law of the Universe (in vipassana, that is termed as dhamma) dictates. I started and ended up making it a practice in my life because I chose it as a spiritual path to really get out of the cycle of birth and death. In the journey of vipassana, I got over many negativities and became a calmer, compassionate and kinder person.
>
> When I look back over the past twenty-four years, I never imagined that the benefits of what I had taken up would impact my life so profoundly and on so many levels, but it has and it continues to do so.
>
> *Shonali Sabherwal*

Here is how meditation will impact and benefit you:

- Definitely reduces stress.
- Makes you less anxious.
- Makes you focused and increases levels of concentration.
- Generates compassion.
- Makes you kinder.
- Lets you sleep better.
- Increases your life span.
- Relieves both physical and emotional pain.
- Decreases addictions.

The following hormones are impacted positively when you meditate:

Cortisol	Meditation controls cortisol with a 50 per cent drop with meditation.[*]
Serotonin	Your feel-good hormone, serotonin, is always up.
DHEA	Individuals who practise meditation have 43 per cent more DHEA than their peers.[†]
Growth hormone	Responsible for repair and rejuvenation growth hormone will help your skin look younger, you will have stronger bones and definitely more energy.
Melatonin	Related closely to the immune function and impacts sleep. Meditation practitioners had an average of 98 per cent more melatonin than people who did not meditate.
GABA	This is a calming neurotransmitter which keeps anxiety under check. Meditation boosts GABA.

How to Meditate

Here is the first technique of vipassana meditation called *anapana* meditation. Follow these steps to meditate:

[*] 'How Meditation Extinguishes Cortisol and Anxiety', www.eocinstitute. org

[†] Meditation and Mindfulness Help Your Hormones and Your Health', www.renewyouth.com, 3 April 2018.

1. Sit comfortably in a posture that suits you.
2. Cross your legs and take a pose.
3. Your spine should be in a straight line.
4. Remove spectacles. Close your eyes gently.
5. Do not breathe from the mouth keep it closed.
6. Breathe through your nose.
7. Focus your entire attention on the area at the entrance of the nostrils.
8. Remain aware of every breath coming in and going out.
9. Breathe naturally and normally. This is all you need to be aware of.
10. If the breath is passing through the right or left nostril or through both, just be aware of this. Do not try to change this. Do nothing. Just remain aware. If it is right, it is right; if it is left, it is left. You only need to be aware. If it is long, it is long; if it is short, it is short. Do not change it, just be aware. The breath comes and the breath goes. Be aware of only your breath. Your mind will wander, but bring it back to focus on the breath and the entrance of the nostrils

Part Four

Guidance from Experts

'Don't limit yourself, discover new areas of expertise.'
—Sunday Adelaja

19

Know and Care for Your Skin

By Dr Kiran Kaur Sethi, MD,
integrative aesthetic and skin doctor,
medical director of Isya Aesthetics,
New Delhi

'Take care of your skin and your confidence will take
care of itself.'

—Amit Kalantri

Here are the major skin types:

- Normal skin
- Combination skin
- Oily skin
- Dry skin

Then there are two adjectives to remember:

- Acne-prone skin
- Sensitive skin

These skin types have nothing to do with your concerns. Whether you have pigmentation, or open pores, or sagging, or acne scars, these concerns are independent of your skin type. It is your skincare that needs customization based on your skin type. I will mention some basic guidelines and common actives used in recommended skin routines, but for a personal skincare routine, do see your dermatologist!

Normal Skin

If you have normal skin, then the skin over your entire face will be even in oil production. You will not have a shiny T-zone and, after you wash your face with a gentle cleanser (not a strong soap or a strong, sulphate-heavy wash), it will not feel dry or oily. Also, if you blot your face with a tissue, you will not see oil or sebum on it.

What Not to Do

- No double or triple cleansing.
- Don't wash your face more than twice a day.
- Don't scrub more than once or twice a week.
- Don't use an exfoliating device more than once or twice a week.
- Don't use excessively foaming or drying soaps, cleansers or washes.
- Don't combine chemical exfoliants like Alpha Hydroxy Acids (AHAs) and retinols on the same day or overdo

the actives without taking any skin breaks. If you exfoliate too much or use too many chemical exfoliants and retinols, you could damage your skin barrier, and trigger rosacea.

The best way to deal with this skin type is to not mess with it too much. If you are one of the rare few to be blessed with normal skin, do not imbalance it with excessive skincare! Sometimes we can get overexcited and push the limits of our skin. If you have normal skin, you have a healthy barrier, and the oil secretion is balanced. If you use cleansers or face washes that are too strong, you could end up with dry skin. If you wash too often, you also dry out your skin. If you use too many layers of products, you can cause acne by blocking your pores. So, the goal is to keep it simple.

What to Do

- Cleanse with a gentle cleanser that is non-foaming or has just a little, gentle foam. If you feel sweaty, then you can consider cleansing once a day with a cleanser for combination skin.
- Choose a vitamin C serum or fluid for your skin that isn't too oily. Avoid ingredients like propylene glycol, as they could irritate your skin.
- Choose a moisturizer that suits your skin. If you like a lighter feel, choose a gel or a light lotion, if you prefer a heavier feel, choose a cream.
- Wear sunblock no matter what. Whether you are outside or inside, you must wear a sunblock! Look for both UVA and UVB protection. I prefer mineral sunblocks because they don't get absorbed in the skin and therefore, better for the skin.

Dry Skin

Dry skin is skin that feels stretchy and tight even if you cleanse your face with plain water. It may or may not have some flaking due to dryness. There is less oil secretion here. People in menopause will tend to have dry skin as their hormones change and fewer male hormones are secreted, which are the hormones responsible for oil secretion.

When you have dry skin, you don't make enough oil. So, you have to avoid things that will strip what little oil you have left in your skin. So, any cleanser with foam or any soap will dry your skin out and pull out deplete the little sebum you have left. Also, if you over cleanse, you will get dry. Scrubs will also dry you out as will retinoids, so be careful with how you use them and how often. Your goal is to protect your skin barrier and moisturize your skin as much as possible.

What Not to Do

- Don't use foaming cleansers or soaps.
- Don't wash more than twice a day.
- Don't scrub more than 1–2 times a week.
- If you are using a retinol, start only 1–2 times a week and then build up.
- Don't forget your sunblock

What to Do

- Cleanse with a non-foaming milk cleanser or oil-based cleanser or just plain water.
- Use a vitamin C-based cream or fluid, or a serum that has ceramides in it or a vitamin C-based oil.

- Moisturize, moisturize and moisturize and look for moisturizers that have vitamin E, ceramides and essential fatty acids in them. Even polyglutamic acid is a great humectant to look for, although it is expensive. Humectant means it binds water in the skin.
- Consider facial oils like rosehip or grapeseed oil which are non-comedogenic (meaning they are unlikely to cause acne) on top of your moisturizer.
- Wear sunblock as the sun can dry you out further!
- Use a hydrating mask 1–2 times a week!

Combination Skin

Combination skin is normal to dry skin on your cheeks, with an oily T-zone. The majority of the population will have combination skin simply because we have more pores, meaning more oil secretion, in the T-zone area. The T-zone is the forehead, nose and chin area forming a T-shape hence it is called T-zone. So, if you use a tissue on your face, the oily droplets will show up only from the T-zone.

People with combination skin tend to think that their skin is abnormal and needs to be fixed. In fact, it is perfectly within normal limits. So, they wash their face three to four times a day, or they use too many actives for oily skin. What ends up happening is, either the cheeks become too dry, or the face ends up secreting more oil to compensate for the dryness created by the products, resulting in further imbalance. Another thing people do is neglect moisturizer. You still need moisturizer. The more moist your skin is, the healthier and younger it stays. Also, moisturizer helps with dehydration of the skin, which is the water balance of the skin. That is independent of how oily you are, which is based on how much oil or sebum your skin secretes.

What Not to Do

- Don't over wash your face. The more you wash your face, the oilier it becomes.
- Don't try to dry out your skin too much—again the drier you make it, the skin tries to create more oil.
- Don't avoid your moisturizer.
- Don't overuse actives for oily skin—you will end up drying it out more than necessary.

What to Do

- Cleanse with a cleanser designed for combination skin.
- Once a day use a face wash with tea tree oil or salicylic acid to reduce oil secretion. It's not needed twice a day because you still have to balance the cheeks which are drier than the T-zone.
- Consider niacinamide serums for the T-zone as they can help reduce oil secretion and serums are easy to localize to a specific area. They don't necessarily end up spreading all over the face, unlike face washes and moisturizers.
- Choose a moisturizer comfortable to your skin.

Oily Skin

Oily skin means that you are creating too much oil in your skin. If you cleanse with water or a non-foaming cleanser, within a few minutes your skin will create so much oil that when you put a tissue on your face, the whole face will leave blots of sebum or oil on that tissue. You will be shiny and oily all over your face. When people are very oily, I always check for hormonal issues in women, as it can often mean the hormones are imbalanced.

What Not to Do

- Don't over cleanse—sometimes if you wash too much, your skin overcompensates and creates too much oil.
- Don't be too harsh with your skin and scrub too often.
- Don't try to treat your oily skin yourself.
- Don't resort to home remedies to reduce this oiliness, they don't work.
- Don't avoid sunblock.

Typically, when people have oily skin, they go crazy trying to get rid of that oiliness. They wash four to five times a day, using harsh face washes or soaps to reduce that oil, and avoid moisturizers and sunblock because they feel too greasy or they are afraid the extra grease could create acne. If you over wash your face, you will actually end up creating more oil because your skin will try to compensate. So, it becomes a vicious cycle! Don't do it! Some of that oil will keep your skin young for years, don't try to remove it all. If you avoid all moisturizers, then again you will not hydrate your skin which is still needed. And if you avoid sunblock, you will end up with a lot more signs of pigmentation and ageing than those who wear their sunblock.

What to Do

- Use salicylic acid or tea tree oil face washes to reduce oil secretion 2–3 times a day.

- If you feel oily beyond that, wash with plain water or use a biodegradable face wipe.
- Look for serums containing niacinamide or tea tree oil to reduce that oil secretion.
- Don't apply more than 3–4 layers during the day or at night to reduce the likelihood of pore obstruction.
- Use a humectant-based moisturizer that is light or gel-like, so it moisturizes without feeling heavy.
- Use a gel-based sunblock designed for acne-prone skin.

The adjectives of sensitive skin and acne-prone skin mean that the skin reacts easily to products and gets red, hot or irritated easily, or means that it easily breaks out with acne or pimples.

During menopause, your skin will change. Your collagen degradation will increase rapidly, so you will start to look older quickly and also, your amount of oil production goes down significantly so that contributes to dryness and also to ageing. Your skin just doesn't feel the same. This is the time to use heavy creams and facial oils to give skin the suppleness it was missing. It is also the time to look for ingredients like ceramides, essential fatty acids, hyaluronic acid, polyglutamic acid and urea in your skincare for improving the skin barrier and increasing the amount of water in the skin respectively.

Therapies like Ulthera will create more collagen rapidly using focused ultrasound waves through a machine that is put onto the skin, in a single sitting, giving a natural face lifting effect that lasts up to a year and a half. While radiofrequency-based therapies will tighten and create collagen more diffusely, they require more sittings—monthly at least.

For deeper hydration, microneedling facials to get deeper into the skin layers, PRP or platelet-rich plasma to rejuvenate the skin, and injectables like Profilho and Volite and Restylane Skin Boosters are recommended where hyaluronic acid is injected into the skin in different ways, and water is attracted to that hyaluronic acid, resulting in deep hydration, collagen and elastin stimulation and more youthful skin. Ultimately therapies like microneedling, injectable moisturizers and PRP will actually make the skin younger, helping you reverse time! In the modern age, there are many nonsurgical ways to still look youthful using skincare therapy in a holistic way.

20

Know and Preserve Your Sexuality

By Leeza Mangaldas,
author, media personality and
award-winning sex educator

'Even in the loneliest moments, I have been there for myself.'

—Sanober Khan

My Pleasure

In my early twenties I remember giving an inordinate amount of importance to a man's skill level in bed. He could have glaring personality flaws; he could treat me badly—but if he was a skilful lover—he'd have me bending over backwards for him. Now I understand that's partly to do with the fact that young men all over the world, and particularly in our country, seem to know so very little about women's pleasure that, when you find someone who does know what he's doing, it can feel like you've struck gold.

But now, in my thirties, and as I hit the ten-year mark as a sexually active being, I realize that it's also partly because of the wildly inaccurate ideas that women inherit about how sex should be. For most of my early twenties I believed that, as a woman, my pleasure was something that would depend on a partner's existing skill level—that if I was to have an orgasm during sex, it would be because he gave it to me.

It took me ten years—TEN YEARS—to realize that my pleasure in bed could in fact depend on MY skill level. That with an intricate understanding of how my own body functions, combined with a willingness to communicate, *I* could be in charge of my orgasms. In fact, I realized the man's existing skill level was almost irrelevant as long as he was enthusiastic and willing to learn.

(I will add a disclaimer here though: unfortunately, for one-night stands and more casual encounters, a partner's existing skill level is, of course, still a major advantage. But if you're going to be spending a lot of your time and mind space with someone, if you're going to be emotionally invested in someone, I've certainly learnt that you should choose the guy who is kind, smart, caring, honest, inspiring and eager to learn, even if he isn't already the best sex you've ever had, over the sociopath who is good at cunnilingus.)

The younger me would also erroneously assume that the quality of my sexual experience with someone revealed something about the level of connection or compatibility we shared as people. If the sex was good, he must be special. But over time, I've come to realize that some people are just very good at sex, like some people are very good at swimming or cycling or dancing. Just because the sex is good doesn't mean that you two are meant to be, or that you share some sort of divine connection. And on the flipside—just because the sex wasn't sizzling the first time, it doesn't mean it can't get better. In fact, by becoming an expert at your own pleasure, you can pretty much ensure it.

As a teenager I had never masturbated. Even after my first several sexual experiences, I thought that having sex was somehow superior, or more legitimate. That masturbation was for people who weren't getting any, an inferior and pathetic substitute. This subconscious shame and distaste around masturbation is hardly unique and comes in large part due to cultural conditioning, but for me it was also from ignorance because I had in fact never even tried. As a result, there was so much about my own body that I hadn't yet discovered. But at the time, I didn't even know that I didn't know the extent of pleasure I was capable of experiencing.

One evening I was chatting at a party with a friend who is bisexual, and she had been seeing only women for the last couple of years. She told me that she had recently had a crush on a guy—but that after getting physical with him, she was terribly disappointed.

'How do you straight girls manage?' she asked incredulously. 'He had no clue what he was doing! I'd forgotten how much guys need to be schooled! I'm definitely not bothering with a one-night-stand with a dude again after this—my vibrator is just so, so much better, and I don't even have to wax my legs!'

I had never owned a vibrator, and I had no idea what I was missing. But if the look in my friend's eyes when she said 'so, so much better' was anything to go by, clearly, I was missing a lot. I asked her to tell me all about it.

'Having a one-night-stand with a guy when you have a dual action vibrator at home is quite literally like choosing to take the bus when you own a Ferrari.' She laughed. 'Even the most highly skilled lover can't compete with the speed and consistency of a dual action vibe!' (A vibrator that provides clitoral stimulation and vaginal penetration at the same time, like the rabbit vibrator that *Sex and the City* made famous). 'It's just a massive technological upgrade from anything a human can do. And it's really taught me so much about the extent of the pleasure my body is capable of.'

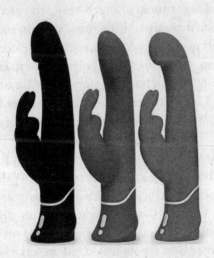

Dual action vibrators

I ordered one online the next day. I will admit it isn't the easiest thing to purchase high quality sex toys in India, but that is a whole other story, so back to the point. The first time I used it, I was so overwhelmed by what I experienced that I thought to myself that if I could make one wish right now, I would wish that it rained dual action vibrators. In that moment I wanted nothing more than for every woman in the world to have access to the incredible depth of pleasure her body is capable of.

I think of my sex life now as pre- and post-vibrator. They feel like vastly different eras.

It was only after I had experimented with my toy that I realized how much more there was to my own arousal and pleasure than I had previously even imagined. And we were only just getting started. Before I bought the vibrator, I used to think that my orgasms were a mysterious and rare occurrence. That it took so much effort to even attempt to get there, that it was so hit or miss, that on most nights I was better off just faking it. Plus, even on the occasions that there did seem to be some magic, it was hard to enjoy myself with abandon, it was hard to stop worrying about how I look and feel and taste and smell, and whether he's having a good time. It was hard to just focus even for a moment on myself.

But alone with my toy, I was able to do just that. There's something about doing an activity alone rather than in front of another person. Consider even an activity as banal and everyday as eating. Wouldn't you eat a bit differently in front of people than you might when you're on your own? And sometimes don't you just want to eat chocolate ice cream straight from the tub, as much of it as you want, without anyone watching you?

It takes a spectacularly high level of self-confidence and self-awareness to do any task in front of another person exactly the way you would do it if no one was watching. I don't think it's any different with sex. My first year playing with my vibrator, I learnt more about my body than I ever had before. Intricately, deliberately, thoughtfully, lovingly figuring out for myself exactly how my body works in relation to pleasure has genuinely been one of the most important steps on my path to sexual self-discovery. I realized that my orgasms are much less complicated and elusive than I had mistakenly assumed, and that I can and should make my own pleasure a massive priority.

The mainstream tells us women's orgasms are tricky, and puzzling, and hard—we're made to believe that for women, orgasms are inherently difficult to achieve. But that's because we're taught that sex is fundamentally about penetration. We're taught that focused and consistent stimulation of the penis is required for sex.

No one mentions the clitoris. If we were taught that focused and consistent stimulation of the clitoris was also required, and that the clitoris isn't just the 'pea-shaped button' at the top, but in fact a much larger organ that extends internally too, believe me we'd be having orgasms just as often as men do.

The full extent of the clitoris

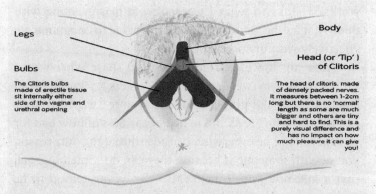

Legs

Bulbs

The Clitoris bulbs made of erectile tissue sit internally either side of the vagina and urethral opening

Body

Head (or 'Tip') of Clitoris

The head of clitoris. made of densely packed nerves. It measures between 1-2cm long but there is no 'normal' length as some are much bigger and others are tiny and hard to find. This is a purely visual difference and has no impact on how much pleasure it can give you!

The "Clitoris" is the entire structure you see here, not just the head or tip of the clitoris that you can see and touch from the outer vulva skin. The body, legs and bulbs lie underneath the skin of the vulva.

Just imagine if we got into elevators without knowing we had to press the buttons, or got into cars without knowing we needed keys, or tried to make rajma without knowing we had to soak the beans overnight. That is literally how most straight couples approach sex in relation to female pleasure—without knowing enough about the clitoris. Penetration alone is rarely enough to make a woman orgasm—which is why most straight women end up having to fake it. Deliberate, attentive stimulation of the clitoris is a one-way ticket to orgasm for many, many women. And a vibrator will show you that—that female pleasure is actually not complicated at all.

I learned more about my pleasure and my body over the first year using this vibrator than I had over all previous years of being sexually active combined. It had literally been a revelation. And as I became better acquainted with the most intimate parts of my body, and more familiar with my own preferences, I also became much more confident and communicative in my romantic life. I've gotten so much better at being able to explain to my partner how my pleasure works. Thanks to what I learned from masturbating with this toy, it has become so much easier for me to communicate effectively with my partner during sex.

After all, if we don't discover and share what works for us, how can we expect our partners to know? And conversely, if like pre-vibrator me, you're swept off your feet by men who are skilful in bed, regardless of how bad for you they might be otherwise, consider this: if the only reason you're with someone is because they can do something well that a machine can do better, it's the wrong reason to be with them.

Don't thank me. It's my pleasure.

Acknowledgements

This book has taken a long time to conceive, prepare, write, format. We first spoke about the book five years ago and decided on a collaboration to uniquely bring together a lifestyle and dietary perspective along with clinical overlay. We grappled with bringing together our two voices and styles and experiences, finally coming up with the holistic view and approach that this book, *The Perimenopause Solutions*, presents.

This book, our labour of love, came to be because of the support of these very important individuals whom we are privileged to have in our lives and for which we thank them.

Hema Malini, for being a role model to so many for ageing gracefully. You have truly been our inspiration as we wrote this book.

Ruby Sheriar, for being our constant support and for keeping us going every time we seemed to flag or hit a writer's block. Thank you for all those trips to Lonavala where the bulk of the writing for this book happened.

Dr Raveendran for being the continued guiding force in Shonali's life. You have inspired much of the lifestyle content of this book.

Dr Rajneet Bhatia and the staff of Aviva Clinic for being the team that backs up Dr Nozer, giving him the space in his busy practice to do all the other things he deems important, such as this book.

Sanjana Banaik, for being there to support Shonali professionally, allowing her to do all the different things she does, all her media work and all the books she writes. Preeti Motwani, for help with all the diagrams in the book. Dr Azmy Birdi, menopause specialist and menopause special skills educator, for her valuable inputs and advice.

Milee Ashwarya, Dipanjali Chadha, Vineet Gill and the team at Penguin Random House India, for their support, extreme patience and professionalism for publishing all those great books for readers.

All the friends and women mentioned in the book for being a part of our work and our lives. Thank you for giving us all those stories to tell and experiences to share that make the narrative in our book special and relatable.

All those women in their midlife and all those soon to reach it. Your perimenopause transitions will bring you unpredictable change. We appreciate all that you have always done for the people in your life. This book is written as a gift for you, and we hope that within it you can find the answers and solutions that you have been searching for, to this enigma called perimenopause

Dr Nozer Sheriar
Shonali Sabherwal

Abbreviations

AGEs—   Advanced glycation-end products
AMH—   Anti-Mullerian hormone
ART—   Assisted reproductive technologies
AT—   Androgen therapy
BHA—   Butylated hydroxy anisole
BHT—   Bioidentical hormone therapy
BMI—   Body mass index
BP—   Blood pressure
BSE—   Self breast examination
BV—   Bacterial vaginosis
CIN—   Cervical intraepithelial neoplasia
COC—   Combined oral contraception
CVD—   Cardiovascular disease
CVS—   Chorion villus sampling
DCIS—   Ductal carcinoma in situ
DEXA—   Dual energy X-ray absorptiometry
DHEA—   Dehydroepiandrosterone

DHT—	Dihydrotestosterone
ET—	Estrogen therapy
EPT—	Estrogen-progesterone therapy
FPHL—	Female pattern hair loss
FSD—	Female sexual dysfunction
FSH—	Follicle-stimulating hormone
GnRH—	Gonadotropin-releasing hormone
GSM—	Genitourinary syndrome of menopause
HDL—	High density lipoprotein
HPO—	Hypothalamic-pituitary-ovarian axis
HRT—	Hormone-replacement therapy
HSDD—	Hypoactive sexual desire disorder
IHD—	Ischaemic heart disease
IMS—	International Menopause Society
IUI—	Intrauterine insemination
IVF—	In vitro fertilization
LARC—	Lang active reversable contraceptives
LDL—	Low-density lipoprotein
LH—	Luteinizing hormone
MHT—	Menopause hormone therapy
MRS—	Menopause Rating Scale
NIPT—	Non-invasive prenatal test
OPC—	Oligomeric proanthocyanidins
OCP—	Oral contraceptive pills
PCOD—	Polycystic ovarian disease
PMB—	Post-menopausal bleeding
PMS—	Premenstrual syndrome
PNS—	Parasympathetic nervous system
POI—	Premature ovarian insufficiency
SAD—	Seasonal affective disorder
SERM—	Selective estrogen receptor modulator
SNS—	Sympathetic nervous system

US FDA— United States Food and Drug Administration
UTI— Urinary tract infections
VMS— Vasomotor symptoms
VTE— Venous thromboembolism
VVA— Vulvovaginal atrophy
VVC— Vulvovaginal candidiasis
WHI— Women's Health Initiative

Online Resources

American Cancer Society
Cancer A-Z
www.cancer.org
American Congress of Obstetricians and Gynecologists
www.acog.org
The North American Menopause Society
The *Menopause Guidebook*
www.menopause.org
American Society for Reproductive Medicine
www.asrm.org
International Menopause Society
Patient education
www.imsociety.org
International Urogynecological Association
Your Pelvic Floor
www.yourpelvicfloor.org
National Cancer Institute

www.cancer.gov
National Institute on Aging
www.nia.nih.gov
National Osteoporosis Foundation
www.nof.org
Royal College of Obstetricians and Gynaecologists
Menopause hub
www.rcog.org.uk
The Hormone Foundation
Menopause map
www.hormone.org
UpToDate
Patient education: Menopause (Beyond the Basics)
www.uptodate.com

Bibliography

Introduction

Baber, R.J., Panay, N., Fenton, A. and the IMS Writing Group, '2016 IMS Recommendations on women's midlife health and menopause hormone therapy', *Climacteric*, 19(2), 12.2.2016, p. 109.

Baria, Zeenia, 'Early menopause on the rise', *Femina*, 2016.

Cagnacci, Angelo and Venier, Martina, 'The Controversial History of Hormone Replacement Therapy', *Medicina*, 55(9), 2019, p. 602.

Houck, Judith A., '"What do these women want?": Feminist responses to Feminine Forever, 1963–1980', *Bull Hist Med*. Spring 2003; 77(1), p. 103.

Chapter 1

Casper, Robert F., 'Clinical manifestations and diagnosis of menopause', *UpToDate*, July 2019.

Harlow, Sioban D., Gass, Margery, Hall, Janet E. et al, 'Addressing the unfinished agenda of staging reproductive aging', *J Clin Endocrinol Metab*, April 2012, 97(4), p. 1159.

Northrup, Christiane, *The Wisdom of Menopause*, New York: Bantam Books, 2012.

Pinkola, Clarissa E., *Women who Run with the Wolves*, Ballantine Books, 1992, 12 and 25–31.

Stoppard, Miriam, *Menopause: The Complete Guide to Maintaining Health and Well-Being and Managing Your Life*, London: Dorling Kindersley Ltd., 2001.

Chapter 2

Guerriero, Giulia, 'Vertebrate sex steroid receptors: evolution, ligands and neurodistribution', *Annals of the New York Academy of Sciences*, 2009, 1163(1), pp. 154–68.

Lee, John R, and Hopkins, Virginia, *What Your Doctor May Not Tell You About Menopause: The Breakthrough Book on Progesterone*, Grand Central Publishing, 2004.

Chapter 3

Larsson, C. and Hallman, J., 'Is severity of premenstrual symptoms related to illness in climacteric?' *J Psychosom Obstet Gynaecol*, Sept. 1997, 18(3), pp. 234–43.

Meeta, M., Digumarti, L. Agarwal, N et al, 'Clinical Practice Guidelines on Menopause: An Executive Summary and Recommendations: Indian Menopause Society 2019–2020', *J Mid-Life Health*, 2020, 11(2), pp. 55–95.

Northrup, Christiane, *The Wisdom of Menopause*, Bantam Books, New York: Bantam Books, 2012.

Novaes, C., and Akmeida, O.P., 'Premenstrual syndrome and psychiatric morbidity at the menopause', *J of Psychosom Obstet Gynaecol*, 20(1), March 1999, pp. 56–7.

Chapter 4

Baber, R.J., Panay, N., Fenton, A. and the IMS Writing Group, '2016 IMS Recommendations on women's midlife health and menopause hormone therapy', *Climacteric*, 19(2), 12.2.2016, p. 109.

Davis, S.R., Castelo-Branco, C., Chedraui, P. et al, 'Understanding weight gain at menopause', *Climacteric*, 15(5), October 2012, pp. 419–29.

Heinemann, K., Ruebig, A., Potthoff, P. et al, 'The Menopause Rating Scale (MRS) scale: A methodological review', *Health Qual Life Outcomes*, Sept. 2004(2), p. 45.

Meeta, M., Digumarti, L. Agarwal, N et al, 'Clinical Practice Guidelines on Menopause: An Executive Summary and Recommendations: Indian Menopause Society 2019–2020', *J Mid-Life Health*, 2020, 11(2), pp. 55–95.

Chapter 5

Baber, R.J., Panay, N., Fenton, A. and the IMS Writing Group, '2016 IMS Recommendations on women's midlife health and menopause hormone therapy', *Climacteric*, 19(2), 12.2.2016, p. 109.

Barnabei Vanessa M., B.B. Cochrane, A.K. Aragaki et al, 'Menopausal symptoms and treatment-related effects of estrogen and progestin in the Women's Health Initiative', *Obstet Gynecol*, 105(5 Pt.1), May 2005, 1063.

Jane, F.M. and Davis, S.R., 'A practitioner's Toolkit for managing the menopause', *Climacteric*, 17(5), October 2017, pp. 564–79.

Krishna, Usha R. and Sheriar, Nozer K. (Series Editors), Krishna, Usha R., and Shah, Duru S. (Volume Editors), *Menopause—2nd Edition (Obstetrics and Gynecology in Perspective)*, Chennai: Orient BlackSwan, 2004.

Meeta, M., Digumarti, L. Agarwal, N et al, 'Clinical Practice Guidelines on Menopause: An Executive Summary and Recommendations: Indian Menopause Society 2019–2020', *J Mid-Life Health*, 2020, 11(2), pp. 55–95.

Mander, Tony, 'NICE Guideline, Menopause: diagnosis and management', *Post Reproductive Health*, 12 November 2015, nice.org.uk/guidance/ng23, 2015.

Stoppard, Miriam, *Menopause: The Complete Guide to Maintaining Health and Well-Being and Managing Your Life*, London: Dorling Kindersley Ltd., 2001.

Chapter 6

Ferriman, D. and Gallwey, J.D., 'Clinical assessment of body hair growth in women', *J Clin Endocrinol*, 1961, 21, pp. 1440–7.

Perricone Nicholas, *Ageless Face, Ageless Mind*, New York: Ballantine Books, 2007.

'Caring For Your Skin in Menopause', *American Academy of Dermatology Association*, https://www.aad.org/public/everyday-care/skin-care-during-menopause

Stevenson, Susan and Thornton, Julie, 'Effect of estrogens on skin aging and the potential role of SERMs', *Clin Interv Aging*, 2(3), 2007, p. 283–97.

Chapter 7

Baber, R.J., Panay, N., Fenton, A. and the IMS Writing Group, '2016 IMS Recommendations on women's midlife health and menopause hormone therapy', *Climacteric*, 19(2), 12.2.2016, p. 109

Barbara Giussy, F. Facchin, L. Buggio et al, 'Vaginal rejuvenation: Current perspectives', *Int J of Women's Health*, 9, 2017, pp. 513–19.

Kim, Jun-Mo and Park, Yoon JIn, 'Probiotics in the Prevention and Treatment of Post-menopausal Vaginal Infections: Review Article', *J Menopause Med*, 23(3), December 2017, p. 139.

Krishna, Usha R. and Sheriar, Nozer K., (Series Editors), Krishna, Usha R and Shah, Duru S (Volume Editors), *Menopause—2nd Edition (Obstetrics and Gynecology in Perspective)*, Chennai: Orient BlackSwan, 2004.

Robinson, Dudley, Toozs-Hobson, P, and Cardozo, L., 'The effect of hormones on the lower urinary tract', *Menopause Int.*, 19(4), December 2013, p. 155–62.

Chapter 8

Arnot, Megan and Mace, Ruth, 'Sexual frequency is associated with age of natural menopause—results from the Study of Women's Health Across the Nation', *The Royal Society Open Science*, 15 January 2020, 7(1), https://doi.org/10.1098/rsos.191020.

Meeta, M., Digumarti, L. Agarwal, N et al, 'Clinical Practice Guidelines on Menopause: An Executive Summary and Recommendations: Indian Menopause Society 2019–2020', *J Mid-Life Health*, 2020, 11(2), pp. 55–95.

Northrup, Christiane, *The Wisdom of Menopause*, New York: Bantam Books, 2012.

Chapter 9

Baber, R.J., Panay, N., Fenton, A. and the IMS Writing Group, '2016 IMS Recommendations on women's midlife health and menopause hormone therapy', *Climacteric*, 19(2), 12.2.2016, p. 109.

de Villiers T.J., 'Bone health and osteoporosis in postmenopausal women', *Best Pract Res Clin Obstet Gynaecol*, 23(1), February 2009, pp. 73–85.

Khadilkar, Anuradha V. and Mandlik, R.M., 'Epidemiology and treatment of osteoporosis in women: An Indian perspective', *Int J Womens Health*, October 2015, 7, pp. 841–50.

Meeta, M., Digumarti, L. Agarwal, N. et al, 'Clinical Practice Guidelines on Menopause: An Executive Summary and Recommendations: Indian Menopause Society 2019–2020', *J Mid-Life Health*, 2020, 11(2), pp. 55–95.

Northrup, Christiane, *The Wisdom of Menopause*, New York: Bantam Books, 2012.

Chapter 10

Baber, R.J., Panay, N., Fenton, A. and the IMS Writing Group, '2016 IMS Recommendations on women's midlife health and menopause hormone therapy', *Climacteric*, 19(2), 12.2.2016, p. 109.

Boardman, Henry M.P., Hartley, L., Eisinga, A. et al, 'Hormone therapy for preventing cardiovascular disease in post-menopausal women', *Cochrane Database Syst Rev*. March 2015, 10(3), CD002229.

Mann, Samuel J., *Healing Hypertension: A Revolutionary New Approach*, Wiley, 1999.

Northrup, Christiane, *The Wisdom of Menopause*, New York: Bantam Books, 2012.

Rosano, G.M.C., Vitale, C., Marazanni, G. and Volterrani, M., 'Menopause and cardiovascular disease: the evidence', *Climacteric*, February 2007, Suppl 1:19–24.

Chapter 11

Graziottin, Alessandra and Serafina, Audrey, 'Depression and the menopause: why antidepressants are not enough?' *Menopause Int.*, June 2009, 15(2), 76–81.

Lovibond S.H. and Lovibond P.F., *Manual for the Depression Anxiety and Stress Scales*, Psychology Doundation, Sydney, 1995.

Myss, Caroline, 'Energy Anatomy—The Science of Personal Power, Spirituality and Health', soundstrue.com, 1999.

Meeta, M., Digumarti, L. Agarwal, N. et al, 'Clinical Practice Guidelines on Menopause: An Executive Summary and Recommendations: Indian Menopause Society 2019–2020', J Mid-Life Health, 2020, 11(2), pp. 55–95.

Mosconi Lisa, 'The Menopause-Alzheimer's Connection', *New York Times*, 18 April 2018.

Mosconi Lisa, *Brain Food: The Surprising Science of Eating for Cognitive Power*, Avery Publishing Group, 6 March 2018.

Northrup, Christiane, *The Wisdom of Menopause*, New York: Bantam Books, 2012.

Thurrott Stephanie, 'The alarming link between menopause and dementia', Considerable, 25 February 2019.

Devi K. Uma, 'Current status of gynecological cancer care in India', *J Gynecol Oncol*, June 2009, 20(2), pp. 77–80.

Chapter 12

'Cancer Treatment & Survivorship—Facts and Figures', American Cancer Society, 2016–2017, 2018.

Meeta, M., Digumarti, L. Agarwal, N. et al, 'Clinical Practice Guidelines on Menopause: An Executive Summary and Recommendations: Indian Menopause Society 2019–2020', *J Mid-Life Health*, 2020, 11(2), pp. 55–95.

Northrup, Christiane, *The Wisdom of Menopause*, New York: Bantam Books, 2012.

Welch, H. Gilbert and Passow, Honor. J, 'Quantifying the benefits and harms of screening mammography', *JAMA Intern Med*, Mar 2014, 174(3), pp. 448–54.

Chapter 13

Armstrong, Sarah and Akande, Valentine, 'What is the best treatment option for infertile women aged 40 and over?' *J Assist Reprod Genetics*, May 2013, 30(5), pp. 667–71.

Auyeung, Anthony, Klein Molly E, Ratts, Valerie S et al, 'Fertility treatment in the Forty and Older Woman, *J Assist Reprod Genet.*, December 2001, 18(12), pp. 638–43.

Harmanci, Reyhan, 'The Truth About Pregnancy Over 40', *New York Times*, 15 April 2020.

Liu, Kimberley and Case, Allison, 'Advanced reproductive age and fertility', *J Obstet Gynaecol Can*, November 2011, 33(11), pp. 1165–75.

Meeta, M., Digumarti, L. Agarwal, N. et al, 'Clinical Practice Guidelines on Menopause: An Executive Summary and Recommendations: Indian Menopause Society 2019–2020', *J Mid-Life Health*, 2020, 11(2), pp. 55–95.

Chapter 14

Baber, R.J., N. Panay, A. Fenton and the IMS Writing Group, '2016 IMS Recommendations on women's midlife health and menopause hormone therapy', *Climacteric*, 19(2), 12.2.2016, p. 109.

Meeta, M., L. Digumarti, N. Agarwal et al, 'Clinical Practice Guidelines on Menopause: An Executive Summary and Recommendations: Indian Menopause Society 2019–2020', *J Mid-Life Health*, 2020, 11(2), pp. 55–95.

Vujovic, Svetlana, M. Brincat, T. Erel et al. 'EMAS position statement: Managing women with premature ovarian failure', *Maturitas*, September 2010, 67(1), pp. 91–93.

Chapter 15

Baber, R.J., Panay, N., Fenton, A. and the IMS Writing Group, '2016 IMS Recommendations on women's midlife health and menopause hormone therapy', *Climacteric*, 19(2), 12.2.2016, p. 109.

Haelle, Tara, 'Change the conversation about hormone therapy in menopause', *Medscape*, 28 June 2017.

Krishna, Usha R., and Sheriar, Nozer K. (Series Editors), Krishna, Usha R., and Shah, Duru S. (Volume Editors), *Menopause—Second Edition (Obstetrics and Gynecology in Perspective)*, Chennai: Orient BlackSwan, 2004.

Meeta, M., Digumarti, L. Agarwal, N. et al, 'Clinical Practice Guidelines on Menopause: An Executive Summary and Recommendations: Indian Menopause Society 2019–2020', J Mid-Life Health, 2020, 11(2), pp. 55–95.

Oakes, Kari, 'Time to take the fear out of the hormone therapy conversation', Ob.Gyn. News, 14 October 2017.

Seibel, Machelle M., *The Estrogen Fix: The Breakthrough Guide to Being Healthy, Energized, and Hormonally Balanced*, Penguin Random House, 19 September 2017.